Truth is not decided by majority vote.

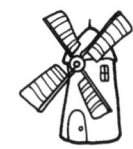

Nutrition and Your Child's Soul

Don Quixote's Heart-Cry

Dolev Reuven Gilmore

Mind-Opening Publications
West Orange, New Jersey

Disclaimer

The author specifically invokes the First Amendment rights of freedom of speech and of the press without prejudice. The information written is published for informational purposes only under the rights guaranteed by the First Amendment of the Constitution for the United States of America, and should not in any way be used as a substitute for the advice of a physician or other health care practitioner.

The statements contained herein have not been evaluated by the FDA. The products discussed herein are not intended to diagnose, cure, prevent or treat any disease. Because of the complexity of the issues discussed, and because there is always some risk involved in using any product or in treating any condition, the author and the publisher are not responsible for any adverse effects or consequences which may result from anyone following any of the suggestions made in this book. And because each person and each situation is unique, the author and the publisher urge the reader to consult with a qualified professional before using any procedure or before refusing any procedure where there is a question as to its appropriateness. Nothing said here is to be construed as advice on whether to take or refuse to take any medication. Some medications can be life-saving. Withdrawal from any medication may result in severe reactions and must only be done under medical supervision.

All statements in this book are the personal opinions of the author, unless attributed to other writers, and are not intended to supplant the personal responsibility of any human being to form his/her own opinions.

Gender-specific words, such as him or her are used because of the limitations of the English language, and are exchangeable. At times, I have chosen one over the other because the majority of those afflicted with some specific health problem may be male or female. At times, the choice was purely arbitrary.

Neither the author, editor, printer, publisher, distributor, nor any related party make any claims concerning the mental or physiological effects of the therapies described in this book, and they cannot accept legal responsibility for any experimentation with these treatments.

First, it is ridiculed.

Second, it is violently opposed.

Third, it is accepted as being self-evident.

— Arthur Schopenhauer (1788-1860)

ISBN: 978-0-9825165-4-6

LCCN: 2009910215

Published by: Mind-Opening Publications
                 21 Greenwood Ave.
                 West Orange, NJ 07052

www.MindOpeningPublications.com

Printed in the Unites States of America

Dedication

In memory of Dr. Abram Hoffer (1917 — May 27, 2009),
To whom a Nobel Prize was due,
In fact, certainly two.
But the windmills didn't reward Don Quixote, either.

To those ill and abandoned, alongside Hoffer's ignored guidance.

To the advancement of true nutritional knowledge,
everywhere and to everyone.

To minds willing to open.

To windmill tilters on all life's paths.

And most of all -
TO YOUR CHILD

Acknowledgements

I've always thought an acknowledgements page must be a most difficult page to get "right." How do you thank everyone? It's so daunting that I thought of being *really* creative and skipping it altogether. Would you have missed it?

BUT, there certainly are some people whose contributions to this book are deserving of mention, so here we go:

My editor, Tzippy Hauser, has been fantastic, going far beyond the call of duty to make this book much better than it would have been had I chosen someone with a lighter pencil.

My cousin and best friend, Devin Satz, who correctly diagnosed the mental deficiency that caused me to start writing this book in a foreign language.

My former student and now colleague, Nadav Alsheich, who changed my spark plug and got me over a serious writer's blockade, while partially authoring the chapter on ADHD.

Dr. Warren Levin, who freely gave advice and inspiration, plus permission to eavesdrop on his letter to President Obama (see Appendix II). Dr. Levin is seventy-something and going strong (*www.warrenmlevinmd.net*). Bless you, Warren.

Frances Fuller, who wrote such a lovely foreword. When I sent sample chapters to her mentor, Dr. Abram Hoffer, he wrote me, "I like what you sent me and will prepare a short foreword..."

Unfortunately, Dr. Hoffer passed away a week later. Fortunately, Frances, the person closest to him in his professional life, agreed to fill the gap.

Christiane Northrup, M.D., for her endorsement appearing on the front cover. I've learned a lot about healing from her books, including *The Wisdom of Menopause* (Bantam, revised 2006), and *Women's Bodies, Women's Wisdom* (Bantam, revised 2006).

Pete Masterson, who did the interior design and gave me excellent guidance in other matters while becoming a long-distance friend.

Michelle DeFilippo from 1106 Design, who did the cover.

Shel Horowitz, who wrote much of the back cover copy and inspired me to do the rest.

Those who gave permissions for quotes and illustrations: The Price-Pottenger Foundation, Pat and Scott Gustafson (Don Quixote painting), Paul Bergner (charts from *The Healing Power of Minerals*), Sarah and Humza Iqbal (poem and letter), Mark Sircus (quotes about vaccines), Victor Kahn (quote from *www.thegreatillusion.com*), William Oeller (Don Quixote woodcut), Chris Neurath, Fluoride Action Network (water fluoridation chart).

Those who read and reviewed and commented and encouraged. You know who you are.

My nieces, Laura and Karen, never far from my thoughts.

My wife, Zahava, our children and grandchildren, without whom my life's colors would be grayscale, or maybe just a watermark.

Contents

Appendices

Foreword

When I first started working for Dr. Abram Hoffer in 1977, I had no idea how profoundly what I learned from him would change my life. The day Dr. Hoffer interviewed me, I was also offered a job working as a ward clerk at a local hospital. Although the job with Dr. Hoffer paid less, I took it because it was close to home and just a few blocks from my daughter Christina's primary school. From this experience, I later concluded that geography — not so much biology — is destiny.

I thought Dr. Hoffer looked somewhat familiar, but I didn't make the connection that he was that Dr. Hoffer: the "controversial" doctor whose public talk I'd attended some years before. Sitting at the back of the packed auditorium, I couldn't see him very well, but I distinctly remembered his response to a question about the nutritional superiority of brown sugar over white. He replied, quite unequivocally, that brown sugar was only dirty white sugar. After I started transcribing patient histories, it became clear that, as well as adding nutrients, removing all added sugar was an important component of his treatment. Then it suddenly struck me who he was, and I was delighted, not so much because I thought sugar was so bad (How could it be? I loved it!), but because I admired his willingness to stand up for what he believed in, and what he had observed with his own eyes, no matter what anyone else thought.

Over the months, what I began to observe in his patients inspired me to learn more about orthomolecular treatment. Chronic depressives, schizophrenics, hyperactive learning-disordered children, even people with arthritis, anxiety, and chronic fatigue – almost to a person they improved or became well on a good diet and the addition of some simple nutrients. Having previously worked in a cardiology office and occasionally "temping" for a psychiatrist, this was a tremendous eye-opener for me, as I had believed the patients' conditions could not be much improved, or that they would have to "learn to live with" their disorder, or take drugs forever, because they really needed these medications.

I also noticed that the people who did not respond, either could not or would not follow the diet (sugar-free and allergy-free), or they "didn't want to take so many pills every day"; and so, they stopped following their program. Clearly, for the best response, patients had to do both.

Curious, I began to read almost every book in Dr. Hoffer's library of over 1,800 books. After his research assistant, office manager, "right hand" and close friend, Margaret Callbeck, R.N., retired, I took over as office manager. Not only did I find my continued reading about orthomolecular treatment fascinating, but I was able to speak directly with patients in the office and on the telephone, and heard from them how these simple measures had helped them. They were also grateful for Dr. Hoffer's encouragement and support. In fact, it was his immediate goal that each patient should leave his office feeling better, and knowing more, than when they had come in. His long term goal was that they should become well. We two became a team, and so began one of the longest apprenticeships in history, I'm sure.

Dr. Hoffer had a Ph.D. in biochemistry, an M.D., and a specialist certification in psychiatry. He helped many thousands of people during 55 years of research and medical practice, and worked for three and a half years as an orthomolecular nutritional consultant. Yet, until his dying day, he never stopped investigating new findings and approaches that could help his patients or clients. He never stopped asking how a condition could be healed or treatment results improved. He never stopped learning, ever – whether it was from colleagues, from conferences he attended, from patients (whose observations he respected), and even from me. He listened to everyone respectfully. He didn't believe he already knew everything, or that he was superior.

After his retirement from medicine in 2005 at age 88, he and I set up our nutritional consultancy, the Orthomolecular Vitamin Information Centre, in Victoria, British Columbia, in January 2006. He honoured me with the title of Associate, and my training as an orthomolecular nutritional consultant began its practicum phase. By that time, we'd worked together for almost thirty years. In late 2008, I began seeing some clients on my own, consulting with Dr. Hoffer after the fact; he always reassured me that I had done as he would have.

Since his death at age 91½ on May 27, 2009, I have been carrying on the nutritional consultancy we started and for which he trained me. Now I'm seeing my own clients, and am ever gratified and delighted when they tell me that they're feeling better and that they're referring their family and friends to me.

What's the point to my introductory history? Simple. Dr. Hoffer was extremely well educated and, for the rest of his life, continued to be informed by his reading, his colleagues, his patients and clients, by his experience and observations. I have a more modest 32 year history of apprenticeship with this great healer.

You, as loving devoted parents, wanting to do your best to nourish your child's body and soul so that she may grow up healthy, happy and fulfilled in every way, may choose to undertake the kind of education and research Dr. Hoffer did, or the lengthy apprenticeship I did, OR you can read and follow this marvellous book by Dolev Reuven Gilmore. He has done the extensive research and reading for you, and has distilled it all into an information-packed (one might say nutrient dense) book, told in a warm conversational style that carries the message without wearing out the reader. You'll laugh, you'll cry, you'll exclaim "Who knew?!" You'll want to make yourself a very healthy sandwich that you can eat while you continue to read. Two little cases out of the hundreds, if not thousands I have seen, and then I'll stop talking, so that you can feast on the book itself.

The first is about a young boy, born around 1970, who had been diagnosed autistic. He seldom spoke or made much eye contact, and he was withdrawn. His parents had been advised to put him in an institution because, the doctor told them, he would never get better, never graduate from high school, never marry, and would never cease being a burden on them. In other words, he was a hopeless case.

Instead, in about 1977 or '78, his mother brought him to see Dr. Hoffer, who put him on a simple diet that was sugar-free and dairy-free, and added optimal doses of some vitamins, primarily B-3, B-6, and C. The boy's mother brought him in several times over the next two years and then we lost track of him. After many years, his file was destroyed.

After Dr. Hoffer retired from medicine, a local magazine published an article about him, including the fact that he and I had established our new business. Soon after, I received a phone call from the mother of this boy we had seen so many years ago. She asked me whether we would like to know what happened to her son. (Of course, of course! The suspense was killing me!)

She told me that her son had graduated from a regular high school academic program (not one for "special" students), had gotten a job and later attended and graduated from art college. He was now married and had a child, and was able to support himself and his family as a well-respected artist. His mother told me that he was quiet and thoughtful, not an overly gregarious type, and that he was normal (perhaps exceptionally so). No one other than his parents, I'm sure, are aware of his former "hopeless" diagnosis.

My second story is about two little girls, both born affected by their mother's alcohol consumption before, during and after pregnancy. They were adopted by their mother's maternal aunt, who was totally exhausted by the task of raising two ill children. The oldest was nine years old and had been diagnosed with fetal alcohol syndrome. She was severely hyperactive, and violent to the point that she could not be left alone with other children, particularly her sister, age six, because she had been so dangerously aggressive toward her. She was a severe school problem, both from an educational and a behavioural point of view. Her younger sister suffered from a milder form of disability called fetal alcohol spectrum disorder. She was less hyperactive and not aggressive, but was having difficulty learning and had social problems, being very shy.

Their great aunt had come to see Dr. Hoffer because she was exhausted and depressed. When she began to improve, she asked him whether he thought he could help these children. He was willing to try, he told her. The girls were referred to Dr. Hoffer near the start of the school year. He concluded they were likely allergic to dairy products, instructed their great aunt how to test for this, and removed sugar from their diet as well. He put the oldest one on 500 mg. of niacinamide with each meal, 500 mg. vitamin C with each meal, 50 mg. B-complex once a day, zinc and omega-3 essential fatty acids. The younger sister received lower doses of the nutrients. Within two months, the older girl had lost her hyperactivity and aggressiveness and, wonder of wonders, she was able to sit still in school and really begin to learn. By the end of the school year, she had caught up to her peers and was near the top of her class. She now had a warm, loving relationship with her little sister, and minded her teachers and her great aunt. The younger girl also was better, able to learn and less shy, now having friends. Their great aunt was no longer exhausted and, in fact, looked ten years younger than her 65 years, as the stress of having to deal with two very sick children had been relieved.

With her two girls, the great aunt moved back to eastern Canada, where they have the loving support of their extended family. We continued to receive updates about how they were doing, both from the great aunt and from her friends on Vancouver Island. When we last heard about them in late 2008, the oldest was 13, a beautiful, healthy, kind and thoughtful young lady, achieving top marks in school. In fact, she was described by her great aunt's friend as a joy to be around. The younger one was also doing very well. All three were well and happy.

The moral of this last little story is really a series of questions. Were they truly brain-damaged from their mother's alcoholism, or were their brains and bodies chronically starved for nutrients? If the damage was permanent, would they have recovered on good nutrition and large doses of nutrients? And finally, if these very ill children can recover completely with the proper use of optimum nutrition and nutrients, how will your darling child improve on an appropriate orthomolecular program? Who knows what potential would be unlocked if her body and brain were optimally nourished?

You have nothing to lose. In fact, you and your child have everything to gain by heeding the excellent information in this volume and following an orthomolecular path to real health.

Be well!

Frances Fuller, President & CEO
Orthomolecular Vitamin Information Centre Inc.
Victoria, British Columbia Canada
www.orthomolecularvitamincentre.com
August 2009

Preface

What this book is meant to be

Informative This book is the culmination of a tremendous amount of study, experience and contemplation. The information brought here is sifted and cleaned of chaff, and I believe you need to know and understand these things. Your perception of nutrition, and how nutrition and our environment affect your children's souls, will be greatly changed by the time you finish reading.

Irreverent, with the qualification that the irreverence is aimed at those people and institutions who so desperately deserve it, and not at the innocent.

Challenging Many of the ideas presented in this book are not generally accepted, even by practitioners of natural medicine. If they were, I would have no reason to write the book. Many conventional nutritional ideas are left out, for the simple reasons that they are common knowledge, and because I agree with them. If I agree with things that everyone already knows, why should I write about them? That's taken care of by writers from the Department of Redundancy Department.

Entertaining and readable I've tried to lighten up the subject matter so that it is readable and will give you a chuckle here and there. Sometimes I think about working up a comedy routine spoofing some of the dumb medical ideas hanging around, and some of the amazing mistakes made interpreting research data.

As accurate and scientifically solid as possible, while discussing subjects about which truth is incredibly difficult to isolate in the sifter. Where technical details are necessary, I have tried to write simply, without sacrificing accuracy.

Lastly, this book is intended to be absolutely head-on, unequivocal, blunt, unswerving, no-holds-barred and uncompromisingly **SERIOUS**. Hello? We're talking about **CHILDREN** here!!!

Some Clarifications

Doctors

I often make rather uncomplimentary statements about doctors. Please know and do not forget while reading, that I am *not* talking about *your* doctor! Your doctor is a dedicated individual who decided to sanctify his life, and gave up just about everything else to study medicine day and night for a major part of his best years. He could have chosen to study law in the daytime and get drunk and something else at night. (Sorry, lawyers, for the insult, but I chose you because you must be used to the jokes by now: "If you saw a lawyer and an IRS agent drowning, and you could only save one, would you have a cup of coffee or would you read a newspaper?") I don't think that most doctors chose their path purely for financial gain. The objects of my "compliments" are institutionalized paradigms, their ramifications, and those who ignore opposing evidence. If any individual is personally offended by my words, please wear the shoe only if it fits.

In addition, institutional medicine can be divided into two major divisions: acute (emergency) and chronic. When it comes to acute medical care — life-threatening situations or when one of your body parts is broken — pleeeease don't ask me about whole wheat flour. (White flour and water make glue, so use that if there's nothing else around.) Modern, Western medicine provides the best emergency care that has ever been provided in the history of the world, saving lives every minute of every day.

Where modern medicine has failed is in the prevention and treatment of disease. The understanding of cause is wrong and the diagnoses are barren, leading to treatment protocols which are wrong. Drugs are given, and then more drugs must be given to treat the side-effects of the first drugs, eventually leading to debilitating emergency situations

> *Professionals built the Titanic…*
> *Noah was an amateur.*

where modern medicine can shine once again, offering several extra years of suffering. One may get the impression that, in this area of medicine, control has been lost to for-profit-only drug companies, to medical equipment companies, and to doctors who have lost their way. The latter have become unintentionally blinded to new or old effective treatments, having accepted a pharmaceutical company's labeled fountain pen while studying a drug-oriented curriculum in college, following that path years later to mandatory CME (Continued Medical Education) ~~golf~~ courses at a Catskill Mountain resort, sponsored by the same company.

It is in this area — degenerative disease — that nutrition is among the most important preventatives and modes of treatment, alongside physical activity and joyous living. Nutrition has been ignored by doctors who use the two letters after their name to claim a monopoly over all aspects of human health. This is the focus of my gripe. An expert should not use his[1] expertise in one area to fool people, including himself, into thinking he is an expert in another. This will only cause damage. Your average doctor knows less about nutrition than does his average receptionist.

For example, I have on my bookshelf twelve books exclusively about vitamin C, one of which I wrote. I have read hundreds of research abstracts, numerous full-length studies and most of what has

---

1   Use of the masculine gender in this book includes the feminine gender and is to be understood as meaning "person." Of course, it goes the other way, too. Use of the feminine gender…

been written in recent years on the Vitamin C Foundation forum.[2] Yet a doctor, who is so ignorant that he never saw fit to dedicate five minutes to the subject, warns my clients that more than a tiny dose of 500 milligrams of vitamin C may cause damage or, at best (wink, smirk), will only enrich their urine with the stuff! Vitamin C is arguably the most important medicine on the planet.

So, individual doctors are not usually at fault, but a system of thought-control which has turned away from healing truth. That's what this book is about — some healing truth, of which every parent should be aware. Sorry, Doc, but with all due respect, you should open up and learn what nutritional medicine, especially the ortho-molecular approach (defined within), has to teach about preventing and healing disease. You owe it to humanity, and to the Inner You, who got you into medicine in the first place.

Soul

This word, soul, expresses many concepts and is understood in different ways in different belief systems[3], including the denial of its existence. There are probably no two people who conceive of the soul in the same way, and most people have more than one concept of what the soul is. I, alone, can describe it many ways:

- The part of a human being that connects to and becomes one with God, in the deepest place. In that place, one soul connects to all other souls.
- The part of a human being that lives on after death, entering body after body throughout numerous lifetimes, carrying with it all the memories, knowledge and experience.

---

2   *www.vitamincfoundation.org* is an excellent and recommended website. I am a regular contributor to the forum discussions.

3   There is an extensive write-up about the concept of *soul* in "Wikipedia, the Free Encyclopedia" on the World Wide Web, for those who want to read how more than a dozen cultures and religions conceive of it.

- The part that is moved by Motown music (seriously!), or any other music, the sunrise (or the sunset, depending on what moves you more), or the smile of a child. And so on, of course.
- The goodness in every person, underlying all his faults. (Sensing this sometimes takes a great stretch of the imagination. OK, in most people.)
- The part of a human being that thinks and feels, and is conscious.
- The source of that indefinable shine, referred to in the saying, "the eyes are the window to the soul."
- The part of a human being that hears, sees, smells, touches, tastes, intuits, thinks and gives rise to actions, resting beyond the mind and physicality.

This vagueness makes me a bit uneasy when using the word soul in the title of this book and many times in the text. I've done enough in this book to offend some people for good reasons, so I don't want to offend anyone for the wrong reasons. The highest divine soul, as in the first description above, has a purity which is certainly not touched or affected by nutrition. So, I am asking for your tolerance here, when I use the word soul to include most of the above definitions, especially the mental and emotional being, the thinking and feeling child, which rests between the physical body and the transcendent. I also use the limited concept that brain function ties directly into the state of this soul, and so it follows that nutrition of the brain is nutrition of the soul, as is nutrition of the heart. Although every physical discomfort or disease affects the soul of this definition, since a sick person cannot be expected to think and feel optimally, we will not be discussing "physical" diseases as such, except as side conversations.

I hope this book touches your soul, as it flowed from mine.

What this book isn't

- This book is not intended to be a comprehensive, a-to-z compendium of knowledge about how to feed your children. Additional study is necessary.
- This book is, obviously, not The Final Word. I invite and encourage you to personally research anything said here.
- This is not a cookbook — for several reasons. *First*, I'm not intimately familiar with kitchens. I swim in different waters. *Second*, many fine books on how to cook healthy foods using quality materials are already available. I've thrown in a short discussion of breakfast because I don't remember seeing cookbooks about breakfast, and because I've had occasion to prepare and serve it to my children and grandchildren, which is the best qualification of all. I also wanted to offer you something practical and daily, since I've been told that people like practical, daily things.
- This is not a total guide to treating anything. The subject is of this book is nutrition, and while I believe that nutrition is *the* primary medicine, other modes of treatment are available for any situation. I will mention some as ideas, but specific treatment must be guided by individualized, professional consultation.
- Finally, as strange as it sounds coming from the author, this book is *not balanced,* though I did my best. No one's opinion can be truly balanced. All of us have our preconceived notions, personal experiences and desires to deal with, and these shape our learning process. If I would claim to have a perfectly balanced opinion, I would be claiming that I know the *absolute truth*. Even Don Quixote admits he doesn't know the absolute truth.

Don Quixote...

Unhindered by the world's opinion, unimpeded by fear. Unbridled by a medical education!!! Free to ride the winds across any field and cast his soul against any foe. The Knight of Good, the Nightmare of Evil. Fulfilling his soul's quest, the dream of his heart's yearning.

Don Quixote is alive — the inspiring, uncompromising teacher, bringing out the best, the absolutely unique part of us, pursuing nothing but pristine destiny, seeing nothing in the world but the moment's highest expression.

They say he was crazy. Well... actually he was, but he got over it. He must have been good crazy, or he wouldn't be among the most memorable and loved fictional characters of all time. Even Mickey Mouse didn't contribute a special word to our language like... quixotic.

Quixotic. Without being quixotic we fall into normality, into everydayness and mediocrity. Without being quixotic, without believing we can conquer giants, we may as well write our epitaph. We would be partially dead, albeit unofficially. Only quixotic men and women can land on the moon and shoot for the stars. Only quixotics will learn to harness hydrogen's energy and harvest the power of our oceans' waves. Only the Don Quixotes of today, the ones who see what millions are still blind to, will guide humankind into a future beyond national boundaries and racial differences. Only the students of Don Quixote will save the children, overcome greed and blindness, and lead the world into a new dawn.

I've heard about Don Quixote my whole life, but never knew that the part about tilting at windmills is hardly a page long. Isn't that amazing? What is it about this one page from a book first published in *1605* that has inspired so many artists and poets and ordinary folk — and now, this nutrition writer? Well, I'll let you decide for yourself. You'll find the page in the Appendix of this book. This picture is the original cover:

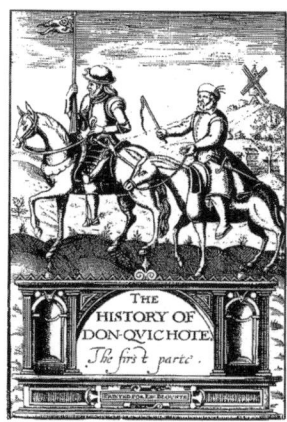

Taking a Stand

Dr. Martin Luther King, Jr. 1967

I say to you, this morning, that if you have never found something so clear and precious to you that you will die for it, then you aren't fit to live.

You may be 38 years old, as I happen to be, and one day, some great opportunity stands before you and calls upon you to stand up for some great principle, some great issue, some great cause. And you refuse to do it because you are afraid.

You refuse to do it because you want to live longer. You're afraid that you will lose your job, or you are afraid that you will be criticized or that you will lose your popularity, or you're afraid that somebody will stab you or shoot at you or bomb your house. So you refuse to take the stand.

Well, you may go on and live until you are 90, but you are just as dead at 38 as you would be at 90.

And the cessation of breathing in your life is but the belated announcement of an earlier death of the spirit.

You died when you refused to stand up for right.

You died when you refused to stand up for truth.

You died when you refused to stand up for justice.

By now, I'm sure you're wondering what Don Quixote has to do with a book about nutrition, doctors and souls of children; and so, let's move on to the Introduction…

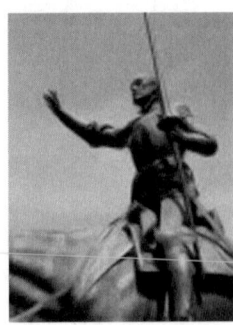

Introduction

Nutrition and Your Child's Soul: Don Quixote's Heart-Cry

I've never really understood what drove Don Quixote to attack windmills, but I, too, know of windmills. I have a demon sitting inside me, poking at sensitive places in my heart and mind, demanding that I raise the flag of battle against buildings stronger than me and bigger than all of us. Although I can't penetrate the depths of Don Quixote's heart and mind, to understand how windmills turned into giants, this suits me, too. Whereas his windmills caught the wind, turning wheat into flour, the windmills in *my* vision *create* wind, wind that covers the whole world with blinding chaff.

I'm constantly amazed by the blindness of the medical world to the importance of nutrition, by the eyes that turn away from what scientific research, clinical observation and, indeed, human history have taught us. How is it that thoughts so simple and obvious have become radical? How is it that experts can miss things precisely at the heart of their fields of expertise? How is it that the public can be led astray by mistakes born of ignorance in matters so central to our lives, such as nutrition? How is it that a mother, driven by limitless love for her children, willing to die to protect them without a second thought, can unwittingly spread the message of the windmills, so damaging to her loved ones?

And just what are my windmills? Tiny institutions like the universe of modern medicine, health departments with numerous branches; little cottage industries like modern agriculture — "agribusiness" — and food producers and marketers; and especially... (and here you may notice that my face puckers up as if I had bitten into a lemon laced with garlic) ...the drug companies. All of these have governmental support and vast financial resources, giving them enormous power to influence minds and shape public knowledge, power which is without bounds. Almost. Only almost, because all around the world there are students of Don Quixote, standing fearlessly by their principles. Yes, there are still pure and innocent souls, who speak up in their purity and innocence, pointing out that the emperor has no clothes, and such things.

Am I making all this noise in belief that I could change the whole world? No. I am not among those pure and innocent souls; I have seen too much water passing under the bridge. A great scientist once said that great changes in the way the world sees things do not come about by convincing people one by one, but because the old people die off one by one, and their places are taken by young people who have grown up with the new ideas. While I'm willing to accept this sluggishness when speaking of great paradigms and anonymous populations, when it comes to individual human beings, "He who saves one soul is considered as though he has saved the whole world!"[4] When I understand that that the person standing before me cannot save himself, that he is incapable of breaking free from his indoctrination, of overcoming his blind faith in physicians who know little about the healing power of nutrition, I feel anguish and frustration. All the more so, when I see those who don't even know that there are questions to ask — the children. Oh my God — the children! The fat children, the autistic, the psychotic, those born with Down syndrome, the hyperactive and those who can't concentrate, children suffering from cancer and all those degenera-

---

4   From the Babylonian Talmud.

tive diseases that our forefathers knew not. For these I cry, and to these my heart goes out!

So the writing of this book, forced on me by the constant prodding of the Lance of Don Quixote, is dedicated to children and their loving parents, and to the many wonderful people, excellent, caring professionals working inside the windmills. They are perhaps unaware of certain breezes outside the walls trying to get inside, and of the chaff that their windmills are blowing into the eyes of the people.

This is a work of the heart, a work of love. Please pray with me that Don Quixote will someday find peace, and will feel comfortable melting down his lance, forming it into a shining jewel.

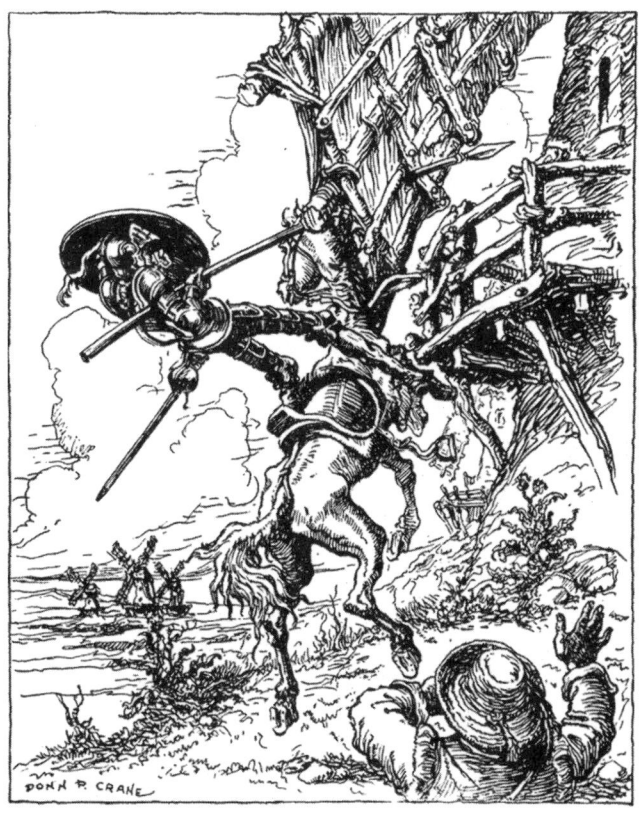

Part One

The Heart Of Nutrition

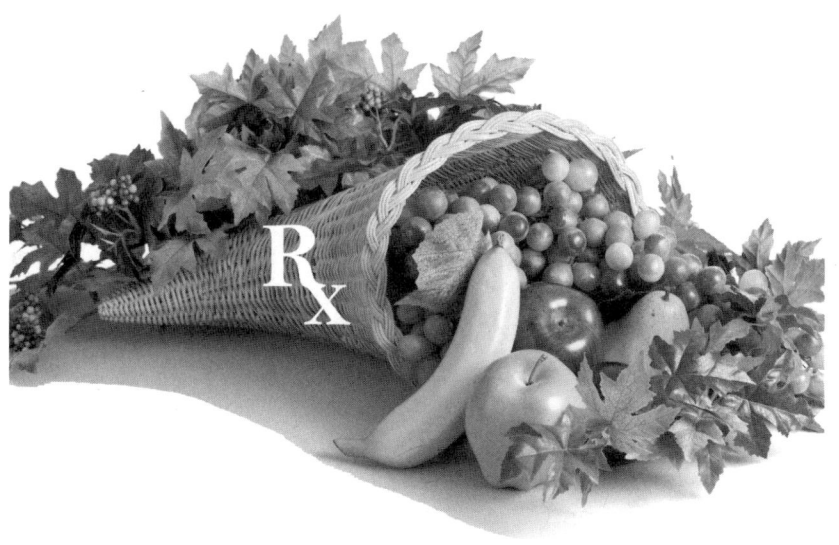

**And Its Incredible Importance
In Your Child's Life**

Chapter 1

Modern Man, "The Wise": Lessons From Teeth

"Each time a person stands up for an ideal, or acts to improve the lot of others, or strikes out against injustice, that person sends forth a tiny ripple of hope... and crossing each other from a million different centers of energy and daring, those ripples build a current that can sweep down the mightiest walls of oppression and resistance." — Robert F. Kennedy

What is proper nutrition, REALLY? Can we get all the nutrition we need for optimal health from food alone, without taking nutritional supplements? If so, how? These are vital questions, and because your family's health depends on finding accurate answers, let's look for some.

The official position paper of the American Dietetic Association (ADA) (*www.eatright.org*) begins:

It is the position of the American Dietetic Association (ADA) that the best nutritional strategy for promoting optimal health and reducing the risk of chronic disease is to wisely choose a wide variety of foods. Additional nutrients from fortified foods and/or supplements can help some people meet their nutritional needs as specified by science-based nutrition standards such as the Dietary Reference Intakes.[5]

The ADA goes on to discuss a variety of situations in which some supplementation may be beneficial. The paper presents a cautious approach to the subject, requiring a high level of scientific evidence before adopting recommendations for specific nutritional supplementation for a specific group of people with specific needs. To the ADA's credit, toward the end of the paper, it opens a window a little bit to the creativity of individual practitioners:

> When do practitioners place their clients and patients at higher risk by not putting into practice newer ideas that have not achieved universal acceptance? Yes, the quantity and quality of evidence must be convincing... However, instead of waiting for leaders in other professions to state their positions on matters involving diet and nutrition, dietetics professionals have the ability to accept their leadership role, to critically assess all of the evidence, and to act accordingly.

Although the winds of change may penetrate this opened window (despite its rather tight screen), the above policies support a conservative attitude toward the use of supplements. Their assumptions imply that for the majority of people, a balanced diet should provide all necessary nutrition, and that supplements are unnecessary.

Every life form draws its nourishment from nature. Plants take what they need from air, rain, light and soil. Animals eat plants and other animals that ate plants. Although none of them purchase or manufacture capsules containing vitamins or minerals, their health is preserved. All necessary nutrients are contained in the food they eat. Man is part of nature. Physically, at least, human beings are no different in any significant way from animals, and therefore the ADA's position makes perfect sense.

---

5   *Position of the American Dietetic Association: Fortification and Nutritional Supplements.* J Am Diet Assoc. 2005;105:1300-1311.

Books have been printed with the king's license,.... read with universal delight, and extolled by great and small, rich and poor, learned and ignorant, gentle and simple, in a word by people of every sort. That these should be lies! And above all when they carry such an appearance of truth with them.

— Don Quixote

We, the students of Don Quixote, know that the rationality of the human mind is extremely limited. People can be convinced of anything. Sometimes, what we accept as true may be a cover-up for the greatest falsehood. The ADA's "best nutritional strategy" may be logical, but the fulfillment of its dictates in the real world — to actually receive all our nutritional needs from a wise selection of foods — is no less fanciful than Don Quixote's attempt to conquer windmills with his lance! To illustrate this, I'd like to tell you about the work of a dentist.

Dr. Weston Price worked in Cleveland, Ohio at the beginning of the 20th century. After a few decades as a prominent dentist, Dr. Price became worried by the increasing number and decreasing age of children brought to him for dental work, by the increasing number of teeth affected by decay, and by the children's deteriorating general health. Hearing from travelers who had returned from journeys to distant lands about the tremendous vitality and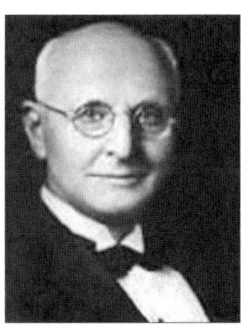

Dr. Weston Price

health of native tribes and cultures, and that the teeth of these people were incredibly white and strong, Dr. Price made a momentous decision. He closed the doors of his clinic and, with his wife, embarked on a quest to far-off lands to personally observe the happenings in these isolated and primitive communities. Dr. Price documented their journey in great detail in one of the most important books about nutrition of all time: *Nutrition and Physical Degeneration*, first published in 1939. (This classic book found its way into my hands only after I had completed a four-year program of nutritional studies. After a half-hour of reading, I was overwhelmed by the feeling that I was being shown, for the first time, the true foundation for understanding nutritional medicine.)

The Prices' journeys took them to isolated villages in the mountains of Switzerland, to Irish and Peruvian fishing villages, to Aboriginal tribes in Australia, to Polynesia, Malaysia and New Zealand, to numerous African tribes, to Eskimos in Northern Canada and to native cultures in North, Central, and South America.[6] Those were the days of the spread of Western civilization, carrying with it modern customs and modern food. It was the optimal time to examine the results of contact between traditional,

Percentage of Teeth Affected by Decay in "Primitive" and "Modern" Populations[6]		
Modern	Primitive	
29.8	4.60	Swiss
30.0	1.20	Gaelic
13.0	0.09	Eskimos
21.5	0.16	Northern Indians
40.0	4.00	Seminole Indians
29.0	0.38	Melanesians
21.9	0.32	Polynesians
6.8	0.20	Africans
70.9	0.00	Australian Aborigines
55.3	0.01	N. Zealand Maori
20.6	0.09	Malays
40+	0.04	Coastal Peruvians
40+	0.00	High Andes Indians
40+	0.00	Amazon Jungle Indians

"primitive" cultures and the modern, "progressive" world. Wherever he went, Dr. Price found some people living according to the old ways, and not far away, members of the same tribe or cultural tradition, already under the influence of the new culture and its foods: whitened flour, sugared treats, canned foods and other products of the budding food-processing industries. Dr. Price examined the quality of the villagers' teeth and evaluated their general health. What did he find? On every continent, among members of every racial stock,

6   Weston A Price, D.D.S. *Nutrition and Physical Degeneration.* 6th Edition. Published by The Price-Pottenger Nutrition Foundation, Inc., 14th printing, 2000. pg. 441. A newer edition is now available.

with no exception, the number of teeth affected by cavities and decay increased in direct proportion to the increase in contact with, as Price himself said, "the white man." It became obvious that the cause of tooth decay, as well as the general deterioration of health, was due to "white man's food." Dr. Price recorded his findings in great detail. The chart on page 34 compares the teeth of people eating their traditional diets with the teeth of those consuming, by will or by force, the products of modern "nutrition."

Bearing in mind that "a picture is worth a thousand words," Dr. Price documented his findings using a tool which, at the time, was becoming quite sophisticated: the camera. More than 150 photographs in his book bring the statistics to life.

Do you see the differences? I'm not only talking about the obvious, the teeth, but about the difference in the vitality and joy of life expressed in these faces. Price found that, in all the cultures he studied, the people radiated health and joy.

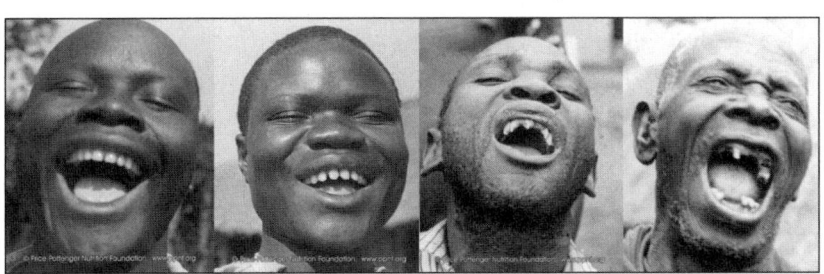

Members of a free African tribe   European plantation workers

He clearly established that the introduction of "white man's food" into the daily menu of traditional cultures was the cause of tooth decay and the general deterioration of health among tribal and village members. Along with tooth decay came other troubles, including tuberculosis and even birth defects. The broad nostrils and wide faces of children born to mothers who consumed the new foods narrowed, forcing the children to breathe through their mouths, rather than through their nostrils. It is commonly believed that life-expectancy among these traditional cultures was short; Dr. Price, however, found quite the opposite. Tribal members remained healthy and strong while reaching old age, continuing to be fully contributing and respected members of their communities. The researcher Stephenson, who had lived for several years among the Eskimos, also reported that tribal people lived long and healthy lives if they survived birth and childhood and then avoided falling through the ice or becoming a polar bear's lunch. If the average life expectancy of any tribe was shorter than ours today, it was because of difficult and dangerous conditions, not because of disease.

Low-carb diet? High complex-carbohydrate diet? How much protein? Low-fat diet? Atkins' high-fat diet? Yes meat? No meat? How many portions of fruits and vegetables? Eat according to blood type? According to your astrological sign or your dominant Chinese element? Yes bread? No bread? Only grapefruit? Vegetarian? Vegan? Macrobiotic? The Zone? South Beach? The Fit For Life combination diet? The newest Wonder-Diet Supplement? How many calories? … etc., … etc… What actually were the diets of the cultures Dr. and Mrs. Price visited? What lessons must we learn from them? Let's look at some examples of their lifestyles and nutrition, before we examine what Dr. Price's findings mean for us.

Swiss Mountain Villages

On page 37 is a recent picture, but the Loetschental Valley must have looked about the same when the Prices visited there in 1931. They found a strong and vital people, sustaining themselves entirely on local produce. The approximately 2,000 people scattered in several villages along the valley had no need for a doctor, a policeman or a jail. Dr. Price did not find a single case of tuberculosis, although it was the most common disease in Switzerland in those days.

During the summer, cattle grazed in the mountains, following the receding snow line, which left lush grasses. While the men harvested hay and rye, the women and children went up the mountains to the cattle, to get milk for cheese and butter. The people recognized the high quality of their milk products, especially the butter. A ritual had developed, which included dipping a wick into the

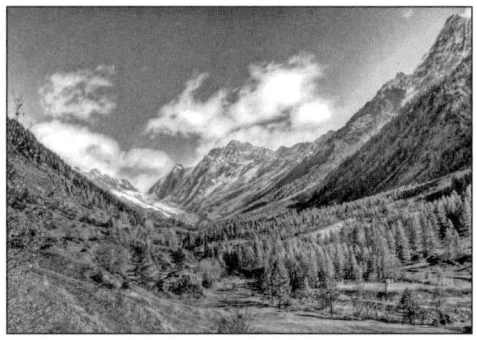

Loetschental Valley, Switzerland

first butter and lighting it in a small sanctuary built for this purpose. Throughout his journeys, Price sent samples of the local foods to a laboratory to assess their nutritional content. Needless to say, these products, even the dried hay, were found to have the highest nutritional value, much higher than the values of today's food.

A typical meal in the Loetschental Valley was based on a thick slice of rye bread with an equally thick slice of cheese, along with goat or cow milk. Rye was freshly ground into flour by hand each day; breads were baked in a communal oven. Meat was eaten about once a week. Among the children, Price found decay in only 0.3% of the teeth, or approximately one damaged tooth in every three mouths, despite the fact that sometimes the teeth were covered with green deposits, because the people had no concept of "toothbrushes" or "toothpaste." These children were so strong and healthy that they would play barefooted in the waters melting from the glaciers in the cool evenings, while Dr. and Mrs. Price wore coats and gloves.

In awe of their honesty and their community spirit of "all for one and one for all," Price wrote:

> One immediately wonders if there is not something in the life-giving vitamins and minerals of the food that builds not only great physical structures within which their souls reside, but builds minds and

hearts capable of a higher type of manhood in which the material values of life are made secondary to individual character.[7]...

When one has contrasted the unsurpassed beauty of the faces of these children developed on Nature's primitive foods with the varied assortment of modern civilization's children with their defective facial development, he finds himself filled with an earnest desire to see that this betterment is made available for modern civilization.[8]

Price compared his findings in the Loetschental Valley to the state of affairs in Vissoie, a village of similar topography. A modern road had been paved to the village a few years earlier, enabling access by cars and wagons, bringing modern food. The people of Vissoie traded their local milk products and rye for white flour, jams, sugar and syrup. A modern bakery was built. Price found that 20.2% of the children's' teeth were attacked by decay.

Australian Aborigines

One clear day when I was young, I realized that the American "Indians" were victims of oppression and greed, and not the "bad guys" depicted in the typical Wild West movie. As I learned more, I began to feel embarrassed about being white. This feeling returned to me in its full glory when I read the chapter in *Nutrition and Physical Degeneration* in which Dr. Price describes the situation of native Australian aborigines. The conditions forced upon this nation offered Dr. Price the opportunity to compare the health of these people in their natural setting to their condition in captivity. That's right, "captivity" is an accurate word to describe the conditions under which of most of this nation lived, forbidden by their captors to speak their own language, practice their own customs or choose their ancient diet. Only a few Aborigines managed to retain their freedom by living in remote, barren areas.

---

7   Ibid. p. 27.
8   Ibid. p. 32.

The food choices of the traditional Aborigines were limited because of the infertile lands with little rainfall which were their portion. From the world of vegetation, they gathered roots, stems, leaves, berries and various seeds. From the animal kingdom, they ate, so to speak, "everything that moves": kangaroo, rodents, insects, birds and their eggs, and fish — when they could reach places with streams. From these foods, taken straight from Nature's table, the Aborigines built and maintained their strong, beautiful bodies. Their sight was excellent, and none of them needed glasses. They could see the movements of small animals from great distances, and proved their ability to see the moons of Jupiter without a telescope. Their teeth had no decay whatsoever, and the width of their dental arch allowed space for their teeth to be straight.

These traditional Aborigines did not fall victim to any of the diseases from which our modern civilization suffers. They were not worried about cholesterol and did not concern themselves with the percentages of protein, fats and carbohydrates they consumed in their daily diets. They were blissfully unaware of the latest Food Pyramid, the Five Major Food Groups or a balanced diet. They were specimens of excellent health, doing nothing more than eating to survive. Not so the condition of their brethren, living in reservations under the supervision of the white man of European origins. Tuberculosis, one of the most deadly and widespread diseases of the time, was rampant among these Aborigines. One enlightened doctor admitted to Dr. Price, that the only medicine that really worked was to send the sick ones to their families who lived the traditional way in distant places.

Clearly, the Aborigines' physical degeneration increased in direct proportion to the distance they moved from their traditional lifestyle and eating habits.

Indians[9] and Eskimos[10] in North America

Fear of cholesterol and saturated fat screams out at us from every street corner, woven into our lives like the fear of children in the movie *Monsters' Inc.* In supermarkets, thousand of products promise to save us from heart attacks and sundry plagues, all because they have 0% or only 1% fat. Vegetable-based products with bright labels assure us that no molecule of cholesterol is hiding in ambush among the ingredients — as if it were possible for a vegetarian product to have any cholesterol at all![11] Even a recent exhibition for dieticians and nutritionists seemed to me a Sanctuary of Honor to the War on Cholesterol in Foods. However, all those who support the idea that cholesterol and fat are a major cause, if not the chief cause, of heart disease, are faced with the difficult task of explaining Dr. Price's findings in his visits to tribes around our planet.

Let's start with the Indians and the Eskimos north of the Arctic Circle in Canada and Alaska. Traveling by small plane, and then boating and hiking a series of rivers and paths, Dr. Price reached wildly remote areas, thinly populated by tribal people who lived as they had for hundreds of years. The long, cold winters, with temperatures well under zero degrees, made it impossible to raise animals

---

9   I do not wish to offend anyone with the politically incorrect use of the word 'Indian'. I have kept the word in the form that was acceptable in Dr. Price's time. Additionally, I recently read that a Native American rights activist uses the word Indian, saying that it is a silly legend that Christopher Columbus called them Indians because he thought that he had found India. Rather, the word comes from Columbus' impression that these people were walking with God (Dios).

10   Here again. I am being politically incorrect in order to preserve Dr. Price's language. The word Eskimo means "eaters of raw flesh," and was originally used as a derogatory term by outsiders. Therefore, the term "Inuit" is preferred by the Inuit themselves. In my eyes, the consumption of raw flesh was very fitting. In the Arctic environment, vitamin C is rare, and scurvy may be a problem during the long winter when vegetation is unavailable. Raw meat contains enough vitamin C to prevent scurvy, which would, however, be destroyed during cooking. When the Eskimos stopped deserving their name because they began cooking their meat, hemorrhagic stroke began to be a problem. This type of stroke is most likely caused by weakened carotid arteries due to the lack of vitamin C, necessary for producing collagen, the binding protein. Additionally, a major reason for the health of the Arctic peoples is the consumption of omega-3 fats, which would also be destroyed by cooking.

11   Cholesterol is only found in animal products. Plants have no cholesterol. Why? One of the many vital roles of cholesterol is to strengthen the cell membrane. Cholesterol is not required by plants for this purpose, because the cell wall is stiff without it. Cholesterol is also the building block from which all of our sex hormones and stress hormones are built. In our skin, cholesterol reacts with light and becomes vitamin D.

for milk, or to grow grains or fruit trees. Tribal nutrition was almost totally limited to wild meat and fish, plus whatever vegetation could be gathered in the summer and preserved.

The health and physical strength of these tribes was extraordinary. No degenerative disease or tooth decay was to be found. Although 50% and more of their dietary calories were received from fat, heart disease was unheard of. More recent studies from the 1970's examined the diets of tribes in Greenland, based on seal and fish, and found that as much as 80% of their calories were from fat, mostly saturated fat! *Yet the incidence of heart disease was a tenth of that of their modern Finnish neighbors.*

In Alaska, Dr. Price met a popular doctor, Dr. Romig, who "stated that in his thirty-six years of contact with these people he had never seen a case of malignant disease among the truly primitive Eskimos and Indians, although it frequently occurs when they become modernized. He found similarly that the acute surgical problems requiring operation on internal organs such as the gall bladder, kidney, stomach and appendix do not tend to occur among the primitive,

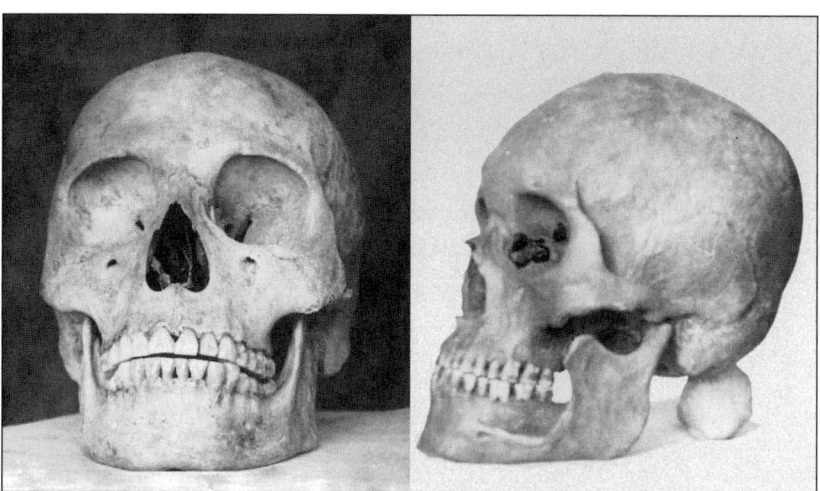

Indian skull about 100 years old. Not only are the teeth perfectly intact, but notice the width of the dental arch, allowing the teeth to be perfectly aligned. These qualities were found in primitive peoples in every place Price visited. However, within a generation after the introduction of a modern diet, the dental arch narrowed and the teeth became crowded, accompanied, of course, by cavities, decay, and tooth loss.

but are very common problems among the modernized Eskimos and Indians... he had seen large numbers of the modernized attacked with tuberculosis... Indeed he reported that a great majority of the afflicted recover under the primitive type of living and nutrition."[12]

Great Differences, Simple Rules

Among traditional peoples around the world, food choices vary according to climate, season, varieties of local plants and animals, and according to the peoples' skills and knowledge of hunting and gathering. In short, they eat what is available. Dr. Price found a great variety of daily menus in the places he visited. Nowhere, however, did he find places that restricted the consumption of meat or other animal products for reasons of religion or health. (He did not go to the Far East or India.) In every tribe or village, optimal health was preserved simply by eating what Nature placed on the table. Except for some cooking, and smoking or drying for storage against periods when fresh food was not available, food was consumed in its natural state. Problems start when we humans get overly clever in our relationship with nature.

We can summarize Dr. Price's findings in this way:

1. Tooth decay is the result of nutritional deficiencies and poor food.
2. Although radical differences exist in traditional diets, they all provide nearly complete immunity from dental decay and degenerative diseases.
3. Laboratory analysis revealed that all the diets were rich in protein, vitamins and minerals, especially fat-soluble nutrients, available mainly from animal fats.[13]
4. In all the diets, there is high nutrient density (explained below).

---

12   Price, ibid. p. 91.
13   The publishers of Dr. Price's book will not allow the use of the book's material by any organization that espouses vegetarianism.

5. The introduction of "industrial foods," as the result of contact with modern civilization, proved disastrous to every population studied.

6. Among children born to parents who consumed refined foods, tooth decay was rampant, accompanied by advanced changes in facial structure — narrowing of the face and dental arch, causing crooked, crowded teeth. They also had more birth defects and increased susceptibility to infectious and chronic diseases.

7. A return to traditional diets brought a stop to the progression of existing cavities, and children born after their parents had returned to these diets had normal, full dental arches.

8. Dr. Price stressed that the survival of humankind demands the application of traditional nutritional wisdom in modern life.

Now we can return to our first question: "What is proper nutrition, REALLY?"
Answer: We need to eat the way they ate.

We, however, live in a very different world with very different lifestyles. Modern civilization, with its wonders and challenges, has changed the world into something those early cultures never dreamed of. We no longer go out to hunt and gather, and our food is frighteningly similar to that which brought destruction to the teeth and health of those tribes and villages. Nowadays, we must ask a new question...

Chapter 2

How Much Food Is In Your Food?

"The trouble with simple living is that... it isn't simple."
—*Doris Janzen Longacre*

The phrase, "nutrient density" appears many times in Dr. Price's book. Understanding this significant concept is basic to the understanding of proper nutrition. We will define it thus:

NUTRIENT DENSITY: *the ratio existing in a particular food between the total nutrient content to the energy content.*

Take 100 grams of white sugar, for example. In each gram of sugar, there are four calories[14] (a calorie is a measure of energy); therefore, in 100 grams of sugar, there are 400 calories. How many vitamins, minerals, fatty acids, amino acids and phytochemicals[15] accompany the calories? How much dietary fiber? According to the database of the United States Department of Agriculture[16], in

---

14   Here and elsewhere in this book, the word "calorie" refers to kilocalories, for the sake of simplicity.
15   Phytochemicals are molecules in plants. Usually, the term refers to molecules giving the plant color, scent, defense or other properties that the plant contains for its own benefit. Many phytochemicals are considered valuable for human health. There are thousands of these whose properties are yet to be discovered.
16   Website: *www.nal.usda.gov/fnic/foodcomp/search/*

100 grams of sugar, there are 0.00 grams of any of these nutrients.

Therefore, the ratio between nutrients and energy, *the nutrient density,* is a big fat (pun intended) zero.

On the other hand, molasses, a raw material from which white sugar is refined, contains, in addition to calories, small amounts of vitamins (not listed here because they are not a major factor in molasses) and a significant amount of minerals, as listed in this chart:

Minerals in 70 grams of molasses (Number of Calories = 155)		
Mg	602	Calcium
Mg	12.3	Iron
Mg	150	Magnesium
Mg	28	Phosphorus
Mg	1744	Potassium
Mg	38.5	Sodium
Mg	0.7	Zinc
Mg	1.43	Copper
Mg	1.83	Manganese
Mcg	12.46	Selenium

Here we see that the nutrient density of molasses is far greater than that of sugar. Molasses can actually be a significant source of minerals in the diet, while being used as a sweetener (after a bit of getting used to the taste). Although one would be unlikely to eat 70 grams (about 14 teaspoons) of molasses in one day, and the high sugar content may make this undesirable, it *is* reasonable to eat 10 grams a day, providing significant and nutritionally valuable amounts of some minerals. In any case, it is a possible substitute for sugar in baked goods and other products. By slowly introducing your children to high-quality molasses, beginning with amounts that are all but tasteless, you can replace part of their sugar consumption.

To further illustrate the concept of nutrient density, let's look at a boiled egg. In two large eggs of 50 grams each, there is the same caloric content as that of 70 grams of molasses, as listed above, 155 calories. We see that the mineral content of molasses is richer than that of eggs. On the other hand, we see that eggs have more fat, protein and vitamins. The protein in eggs is considered to be of the highest quality, a complete protein, since it contains all of the essential amino acids (the building blocks of proteins). An egg even contains phytochemicals, the amounts and types of which are dependent on the diets of the chickens that laid the eggs.

From this table, we can conclude that the nutrient density of an egg is greater than that of molasses, despite the fact that it's impossible to come up with an exact number. Of course, each food type has its own nutritional purpose. If, for example, I would like a client to increase their intake of potassium, I could recommend using molasses as a sweetener, in place of white or brown sugar. If they suffer from general malnutrition, or if their cholesterol is too low (yes, there most certainly *is* such a thing), then I could recommend eating a couple of eggs each day.

Boiled Egg – 100 Grams (155 Calories)		
Protein	12.6	grams
Fat	10.7	grams
Cholesterol	424	Mg
Vitamins		
A	5869	I.U.
E	1.03	Mg
K	0.3	Mcg
B12	1.1	Mcg
Folic acid	44	Mg
Minerals		
Calcium	50	Mg
Iron	1.19	Mg
Magnesium	10	Mg
Phosphorus	172	Mg
Potassium	126	Mg
Sodium	124	Mg
Zinc	1.05	Mg
Copper	0.01	Mg
Manganese	0.03	Mg
Selenium	30.8	Mcg

The important thing about the concept of nutrient density is not the specific details in the charts, but the general idea. Just as the populations studied by Dr. Price were not guided by the Food Pyramid when choosing their foods, they also did not calculate their nutrient consumption according to Department of Agriculture charts. They simply ate from the table that Nature spread before them. They ate nutrient-dense foods, a concept worth internalizing.

There are further limitations when using food data charts. We mentioned that Dr. Price continually sent samples of foods to the laboratory for analysis. He found that the food samples he sent were of greater nutritional value than their "modern" counterparts. Loetschental Valley butter is not at all comparable to the butter we buy today. The quality of organic eggs from free-range chickens, readily available today, is far greater than that of eggs from chickens raised three to a small cage and fed only grain. The values in food data charts are not etched in stone. The nutritional content of a particular food changes according to the quality of the soil in which it grew and according to the particular variety of the plant, as well as many other influences. Food charts can not relate to these factors.

However measured, modern food cannot be compared to the food eaten by the primitive tribes and in traditional villages. Leaving aside the damaging junk foods sold to us by food industries that have no regard for anything but profits, even most of our "good" food is lacking and inferior. Why? Here are a few reasons.

Modern Industrialized Agriculture (Agribusiness)

Every atom and molecule we eat enters our food from the environment — from the earth, through plants. We eat the plants directly, or we eat animals that ate plants. In the forest life-cycle, what a plant takes up from rich forest earth and internalizes goes back into the forest floor when the plant dies and naturally composts, or in the form of animal droppings, dead animals or microorganisms which live on plant material. Forest life is rich, and the great variety of life in all forms sustains itself indefinitely.

In stark contrast, following the "wise" dictates of "progressive" agriculture, a single type of plant is grown year after year in the same large field, accompanied — when done successfully and properly, of course — by the destruction of all other plant life, animal life and even microorganism life in the soil. Using a wide variety of chemicals, the "growing medium" is "purified." After the favored plant draws its sustenance from the earth, it is cleared off — sometimes only its fruit or seed, sometimes completely. In this way, the plant's nutrients are drawn from the earthly stores and, if they are not replaced, the ground becomes nutrient-deficient.

Using a theoretical example and simple arithmetic, let's illustrate the problem of caring for the earth so that it properly feeds the plants that feed us. Imagine a new essential nutrient called "alph," which is like a new mineral. If we measure the amount of alph in an acre of land, we would find that there are 2000 grams in that acre, down to the depth of one yard, which happens to be the depth which the roots of an imaginary plant, the "motambo," reach. When we harvest our acre of motambo, we receive a yield of 1000 pounds. Chemical analysis shows that each pound contains 200 milligrams of alph. A quick calculation reveals that a total of 200 grams of alph were absorbed from the earth by the motambo, leaving 1800 grams of alph in the field.

It is easy to see that within a few years of mono-cropping motambo, there will be a serious decline in the reservoir of alph available for future generations of motambo. Motambo will absorb less alph year after year. This deficiency can show up in two ways. Either the plant will not grow well because it needs alph to do so, or it will grow well anyway, but will have less alph in it for the benefit of the people who will consume it. These consumers may then have a nutritional deficiency of alph, which may have far-reaching effects on their health. (This deficiency, according to the system of the windmills, will be treated by a poisonous drug, which will create side affects that will be treated with other drugs... rather than being treated by simply supplementing the diet with alph.)

What did we, Homo sapiens (which means, "Man, the wise," a nickname given to us by us, not by motambos or by apes), learn to do in order to treat this problem of continual depletion of nutrients? The answer is simple. We fertilize the ground, in an attempt to mimic the Ways of the Forest Floor. When we fertilize with plenty of organic materials, like manure or compost, there is a decent chance that we will more or less replace what was drawn out by the previous crop. Perhaps we will even improve the soil beyond it's original nutritional state. However, the common chemical fertilizers used by agribusiness contain only those elements needed to make a plant give a good *yield* — usually nitrogen, potassium and phosphorus. No thought is given as to the nutritional value of that plant when it reaches our plates. Therefore, in our food today — even in healthy foods like fruits and vegetables — there is a deficiency of minerals and other important nutrients. This is a representative chart of what has happened over time, with statistics from the U.S. Department of Agriculture. The famous "Apple a day" will no longer "keep the doctor away," having lost most of its vitamin and mineral content:

AN APPLE A DAY... The receding nutritional value of an apple from generation to generation				
MINERALS (Mg)	**1914**	**1963**	**1992**	**% CHANGE (1914-1992)**
CALCIUM	13.5	7.0	7.0	- 48.15
PHOSPHORUS	45.2	10.0	7.0	- 84.51
IRON	4.6	0.3	0.18	- 96.09
POTASSIUM	117	110	115	- 1.71
MAGNESIUM	28.9	5	5	- 82.7
VITAMINS	**1914**	**1963**	**1992**	**% CHANGE**
A (I.U.)		90	53	- 41.11
C		4	5.7	+ 42.503
B1	No Data[17]	.03	.017	- 43.33
B2		.02	.014	- 30.00
B3		0.1	.077	- 23.00
				Source: USDA, 1963 and 1997

Our meat is also very, very different from the meat our predecessors ate. This chart compares the nutritional value of modern barn-raised, grain-fattened beef to the meat of wild deer and range-fed bison.[18]

Nutrients in Domestic Beef vs. Wild Game (100 Grams)				
Nutrient	**Beef**	**Deer**	**Bison**	**% Change**
Fat	19.2	2.42	1.84	+ 534
Essential fats	3.59	15.7	7.61	- 68
Iron	1.85	3.4	2.6	- 22.6
Magnesium	19	23	25	- 24
Potassium	297	318	343	-18
Copper	0.07	.025	0.09	- 61
Manganese	0.01	0.04	0.01	- 37

---

17 In 1914, vitamins were just being discovered, so there is no data as to their content in food.
18 Source: USDA, 1997. From Bergner, p. 39.

Note that although there is more than five times the amount of fat in domestic beef compared to wild meat, there are considerably less *essential* fats — less than half — in domestic beef. This is very unhealthy. Even among the cultures that consumed a larger proportion of their calories from meat than we do, the fat's composition — the percentages of the various saturated and unsaturated fatty acids — was much more beneficial for health. These essential fatty acids include the "omega-3" family, so very important for the soul of your child. (We will discuss them at length later on.) Omega-3 is found in the grasses of the field; very little reaches the meat of animals raised at the feeding trough. Even in places where a calf is allowed to eat grass alongside its mother on the open range, in most cases, it is locked up in a small pen and stuffed with grain for a few months before slaughter. There, the amount of omega-3 in its flesh drops drastically, as illustrated in this graph.

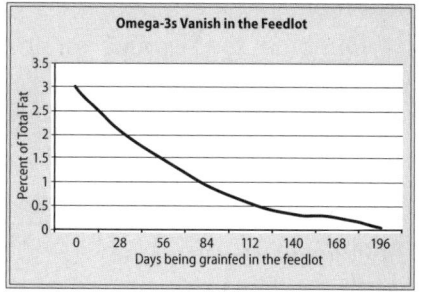

All tribal cultures recognized the importance of eating meat from the pasture or the hunt. I once met an Israeli man of Ethiopian descent, who described his life in a remote village before moving to Israel. His description of his childhood village could have been a chapter in Dr. Price's book. He told me that, even now, he and several family members travel for three hours to cattle ranches in the Golan Heights, where they purchase a calf directly from the pasture and divide up the meat. In the United States, and in many other countries, range-fed meat is available in select health food stores, and can even be purchased through the Internet. Sometimes, the price difference is not large, and the investment will repay itself in the health of your family.

Modern agribusiness also feeds us foods contaminated with pesticides, herbicides, hormones, antibiotics and probably more types of chemicals than we ever imagined — all of which are foreign to our bodies. Besides the damage of directly poisoning the wondrous and delicate biochemical processes in our bodies, additional damage is caused by the fact that our bodies must allocate valuable nutritional resources to neutralize and excrete these chemicals, and to repair the damage they do. One example is vitamin C. Having reviewed thousands of studies about this vitamin, it is my personal opinion that the doses which were found effective forty or fifty years ago are often no longer as effective today. Vitamin C neutralizes an incredible number of modern environmental poisons[19]. The small amounts of this vitamin we receive from food are "wasted" for this noble purpose, even before they can be used in fundamental bodily processes. Supplemental vitamin C is necessary for the optimal health of all modern people.

Our other food groups are similarly damaged. Milk products from the modern cow, living in her own excretions and eating grain, cannot be on the same health-giving level as products made from the milk of cows pastured in the Swiss Alps. Eggs from chickens raised three or four in a cage, in vast lines of cages, are not... Well, at least organic eggs nowadays are of high quality. Buy them — they are worth the extra money.

The Food Industry

Removing parts of seeds and grains — such as wheat bran and wheat germ — and grinding the remainder into white flour, refining vegetable oils, processing sweet plants to leave only their white, simple sugar content, preserving fruit in syrup and as jam, pasteurizing and homogenizing milk, the war against fat, genetically modifying foods (Improving?? Don't make me laugh!), adding synthetic colors, tastes, emulsifiers, sweeteners, preservatives, anti-caking agents, stabilizers, thickeners and God knows what else — all this damages the quality of the food we eat, and therefore damages overall public health. Is it necessary? Perhaps. Perhaps some of these things are necessary, but

---

19   The best book on this subject is *Vitamin C, Infectious Diseases, and Toxins*, by Dr. Thomas Levy.

they are still harmful. The chart below illustrates what happens to the nutritional value of bread when we favor *our* wisdom and taste buds over the wisdom of nature, when we make white bread, "fit for kings":

Nutritional Value: White Bread vs. Whole Wheat Bread (100 grams)			
Nutrient	Whole Wheat	White Bread	% Difference
Protein	9.5	8.9	- 6.3
Fat	1.5	0.6	- 60
Fiber	1.5	0.1	- 93.3
Minerals			
Calcium	25	10	- 60
Iron	2.5	1	- 60
Magnesium	86	24	- 72
Phosphorus	229	94	- 60
Potassium	250	65	- 74
Zinc	1.94	0.62	- 68
Copper	0.284	0.125	- 56
Manganese	2.32	0.383	- 83.5
Vitamins			
Thiamin B1	0.27	0.08	- 70
Riboflavin B2	0.1	0.04	- 60
Pyridoxine B6	0.179	0.064	- 64
Folic Acid mcg	50	34	- 32
E International Units	6.0	0.19	- 97

Contemplate this chart and ask yourself: "How will the constant consumption of white bread affect the physical health and the soul of my child?" Many parents, suffering from financial distress, do not, or cannot, allow themselves to purchase whole wheat bread, which can cost twice as much as white bread. The table clearly indicates that the nutritional value of white bread can be less than half that of whole wheat bread. Since the number of calories in the two types of bread is very close, we can clearly understand the tremendous gap in the all-important nutrient density. *You actually get more than your money's worth of nutrition when you pay more for the whole-grain bread!* Additionally, when you begin to purchase whole-grain, healthy breads for your family, you will also notice that less is eaten. White bread fills the belly without giving a feeling of satisfaction — or at least the satiety will be short-lived. Empty calories from foods with low nutrient density will not provide health and satisfaction. These calories are just sugars. The lower cost of white bread is just an illusion, a very profitable one for those windmills, the ones that raise the wrath of my teacher, Don Quixote.

What is this "War Against Fat," and why did I include it in my list of damages caused by the food industry? Don't fats and especially cholesterol harm us and make us fat? Don't they cause heart attacks? If so, we *should* declare war against their consumption, except where unavoidable. Here again, dear readers, we run into one of those generally accepted concepts about which it may be advisable to raise some very serious doubt. Did we not see that among the cultures visited by Dr. Price, animal products were eaten in quantities, and the fat content was valued? Those people lived without heart disease and the degenerative diseases that afflict our modern society. Of course, we cannot say that the fact that they ate animal fats is the cause of their good health, since there are many other differences between their lifestyles and ours. They had much more exercise, for one thing. However, even if eating fat may possibly not be the *cause* of their good health, it certainly did them no *harm*! So why should we take it for granted that fat harms us?

We will refrain from a long dissertation about how it came about that our minds and opinions have been influenced to believe what we believe about fats. This is beyond the scope of this book, which is, after all, a book about how nutrition affects the soul of a child. Let it suffice to quote Don Quixote, when asked this question by one of us students:

"The answer, my dear friends, is to be found not in the fields of science and medicine, but in the fields of politics and economics, those fields occupied by... WINDMILLLLS!!!"

Here is one final chart, illustrating the diminished nutritional value of low-fat products. Is it worth it to lower the fat content of natural foods at the price of lowering their nutritional value?

Cheddar Cheese: Whole vs. Low-Fat			
Nutrient	Whole	Low-Fat	% Difference
Protein	24.9	24.35	2 -
Fat	33.1	7	79 -
Calcium	721	415	43 -
Potassium	368.4	66	82 -
Iron	0.68	0.42	38 -
Zinc	3.11	1.82	42 -
Copper	0.031	0.021	32 -
Manganese	0.01	0.006	40 -
Vitamin A	1059	233	78 -
Vitamin E	0.24	0.08	67 -

Dr. Price's classic work, described in elegant detail in his book, *Nutrition and Physical Degeneration,* can be summarized succinctly and unambiguously: most disease arrives not from our genes, not from viruses or bacteria, not from cholesterol and fats, not idiopathically (a fancy medical word meaning, "we have no idea what causes it"), not from outer space, or by the wrath of God or by chance — but from our table, from the physical degeneration caused by our faulty nutrition and modern lifestyle.

Let's not forget the question we asked at the beginning of Chapter One: Do we need nutritional supplements, or can we receive all the nutrition we need from food only? The answer of the Dietetics Association, a stance generally accepted and espoused by various branches of conventional medicine, would be: "Certainly, for most of the general population." This opinion looms before my eyes just as a windmill stood before the eyes of Don Quixote. As Don's sworn disciple, I cannot resist the urge to attack. What is most frustrating and maddening is that the words they use are correct. It's as if you were to tell me that a kilogram of gold is on the roof of a three-story building, and that the gold is mine, on the condition that I jump up there without mechanical assistance. I simply cannot do it. In the same manner, yes, in *theory*, you *can* get all your nutritional needs from a balanced diet, but, in the real world today, you simply can't. You know what? You can try, and *even* succeed, if you follow 14 "simple" rules. Post this on your refrigerator:

I Can Get All The Nutrition Necessary For My Family's Optimal Health From Food Alone If I Follow:

The Fourteen Rules

1. Eat only organic produce, including some wild plants.
2. Use only whole grains and flours.
3. Eat only organic, not "regular," eggs from free-range chickens.
4. Use only fresh, whole milk products that have not undergone pasteurization or homogenization, from cows raised according to the natural, "organic" system of agriculture, mainly eating in pastures.
5. Consume plenty of essential fatty acids at a ratio of omega-6 to omega-3 of not more than 4 to 1.
6. Eat meat only from range-fed or wild animals.
7. Completely avoid consumption of simple sugars.
8. Completely avoid consumption of margarine, hydrogenated and partially hydrogenated fats and refined oils.
9. Completely avoid the use of street drugs, prescription drugs and medicines (including contraceptive pills).
10. Live a lifestyle that includes varied exercise and lots of it.
11. Stay completely healthy, and especially, have no problems of digestion and absorption.

[handwritten note in left margin:] #2 Questionable not suitable for very thin people or weak digestion

12. Live in a completely pure and non-polluted environment.
13. Drink pure water, from a source far from "the white man."
14. Live with joy and happiness, satisfaction and self-realization, in a loving personal environment, a life without chronic stress.

"Not simple? So follow each rule the best you can and take supplements," says Don Quixote.

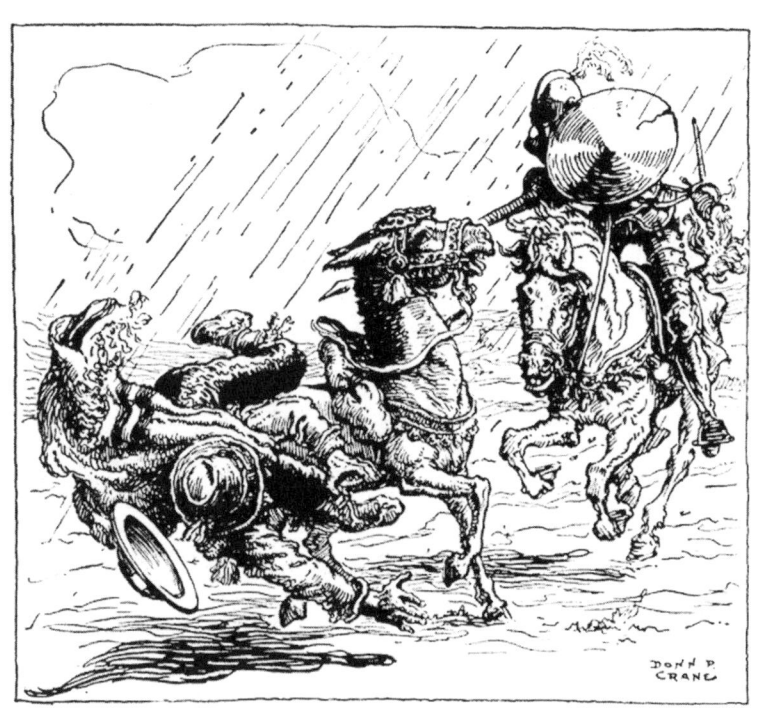

Chapter 3

The Two Faces of Malnutrition

To see our children succeed in school is a wish and hope we all share. Abundant human and financial resources are invested toward this goal by all government education and social welfare agencies, and by individuals involved in education. New books are constantly being published, applying the newest educational theories; teachers attend continuing education programs; children having difficulty learning are placed in special programs, art therapy and music therapy. There is a psychologist in every school, drugs are used (Don Quixote's ears just perked up), and endless efforts are made to improve our children's learning skills. Nutrition, as a means of improving learning abilities, is given much less respect than it deserves. Serious consideration of nutritional supplements is completely absent. In this chapter, we will discuss the influence of nutrition on the learning ability and behavior of relatively *healthy* children.

At what point does faulty nutrition cause the brain to cease functioning optimally? The extremes are clear: everyone will agree that the brain functions best when nutrition is optimal, however we define "optimal." I also assume that everyone would agree that the brain functions at its worst when the person carrying this brain in his head dies of hunger. If we sketch a graph, how would the line describing brain function between these two extremes appear? Does brain function remain optimal in the face of minimal nutritional deficiencies until they become severe, and then drop drastically?

This is described by the dashed line on the chart. Or perhaps the decline in brain function begins with even a slight nutritional deficiency, as described by the light, diagonal line, a decline in direct relationship to the decline in nutritional quality. In

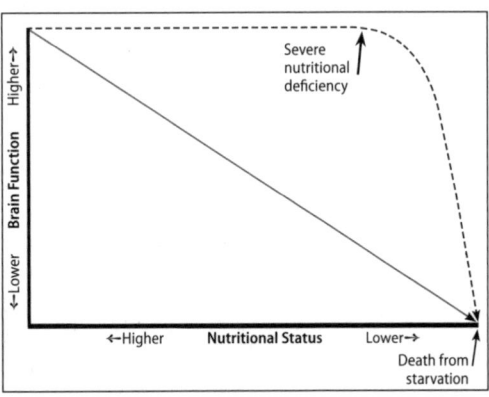

other words, is the expression of our children's souls in the world damaged by the consistent nutritional deficiencies, the fruits of our modern windmills, which assure that their rightful quota of nutrients will never reach the table? So as not to keep you in suspense any longer, I have recorded Don Quixote's answer for you: **"Yeessss!!!"** he shouts, and his powerful voice echoes along the canyon walls.

In several American schools, an amazing transformation in student behavior took place after nutritional improvements were made in the cafeteria. In Appleton, Wisconsin, fast-food hamburgers and fries on a bun were replaced by meats prepared from home recipes, fresh fruits and vegetables, and whole wheat bread. Water replaced sweetened drinks, and vending machines selling junk food disappeared from the hallways. The results? Grades improved, there were less arguments and, as one teacher said, "I can now spend my time teaching, rather than in disciplining." Other quotes from teachers and administrators:

> I've taught here almost 30 years. I see the kids this year as calmer, easier to talk to. They just seem more rational...
>
> Dropouts are non-existent. Kids came to school. They have learned that with healthier foods it's going to make them a better person. It keeps them more focused and makes them happier.

I don't have the angry outbursts, so instead we get to deal with the real issues... (school psychologist)

We have not had one incident all year that I have had to get involved in with shoving, a fight, aggressive behavior.

Finally, as one student said, "Now I can concentrate better and think more clearly. I think I get along with people better. What a revelation: eating healthier food improves concentration and thinking!"

Many schools make deals with soft drink distributors and profit from the sales of sweetened, colored drinks (read "dirty water"), at the expense of the children's health and spiritual well-being. In one typical can of drink, ten teaspoons(!) of sugar (4 grams per teaspoon) are hidden, not to mention sundry other chemicals. How many cans does your child drink each day? Many children drink four cans or more every day, which means they are consuming, just from drinks, 40 teaspoons = 160 grams = more than ⅔ of a cup of sugar a day! This comes out to nearly 2½ pounds of sugar a week — and that is only from drinks!!! (The background noise you hear is Don Quixote simply wailing in anguish.) Artificial sweeteners are problematic in their own way[20], so "Diet" drinks are no better. Sweetened drinks are the largest source of simple sugars in the American diet.[21] Simply eliminating them from your child's life will immediately improve his physical and mental functioning, as well as his prospects for living a worthwhile life.

> "The drink of the wise man is water."
> — Chinese saying

Many research projects have taught us about the benefits of a healthy breakfast. Children who eat a typical breakfast with low nutrient density, or who skip breakfast entirely, react more slowly to mental stimulus. Their memory is damaged, and their scores on

---

20   See chapter 13.
21   American Journal of Clinical Nutrition 1995: 62: 178S-194S.

cognition and creativity tests are lower.[22,23] It has also been demonstrated that a good breakfast improves the behavior and social relationships of children of all ages, as well as lowering absenteeism and expulsions from school.[24] In a very interesting study, most students who participated in a school breakfast program felt that the breakfast improved their energy levels and helped them concentrate.[25] These children were less worried about their weight, in comparison to those who did not participate in the program.[26] One scientist summarized his examination of the research on how breakfast affects children: "...available information suggests that brain function is sensitive to short-term variations in the availability of nutrient supplies."[27] Of course that's true — the brain is an organ just like any other organ, and every organ needs nutrients constantly. In fact, the brain's use of nutrients is greater than that of any other organ, in relation to size.

All of the findings in the last paragraph are true, even among children who are not recognized as suffering from malnutrition. Among children who are in greater danger of malnutrition, generally from families whose level of income places them below the poverty line, the statistics stand out even more clearly. All problems of learning, behavior and emotional instability are understandably worse in hungry children, particularly aggressiveness and nervousness.[28] Teachers have reported increased incidence of hyperactivity, tardi-

22   *Fasting and cognition in well and undernourished schoolchildren: a review of three experimental studies.* E. Pollitt, S. Cueto, E.R. Jacoby. American Journal of Clinical Nutrition, 67(4): 779S 784S. 1998.
23   *An experimental study of the effects of energy intake at breakfast on the test performance of 10 year old children in school.* D.P. Wyon, et al. International Journal of Food Sciences and Nutrition, 48(1): 5 12. 1997.
24   *Breakfast and Performance.* S. Cueto. Public Health Nutrition, 4(6A): 1429-31. 2001.
25   *Children's perceived benefits and barriers in relation to eating breakfast in schools with or without universal school breakfast.* J. Reddan, K. Wahlstrom, M. Reicks. Journal of Nutrition Education and Behavior, 34: 47-52. January/February 2002.
26   Ibid.
27   *Does breakfast make a difference in school?* E. Pollitt. Journal of Amer. Dietetic Assn., 95(10): 1134 1995.
28   *Hunger in children in the United States: potential behavioral and emotional correlates.* R.E. Kleinman. Pediatrics, 101(1): E3. 1998.

ness and absence among these children.29 Particularly worrying is research that points to the fact that malnutrition in the early years of life can negatively affect scholastic achievements years later. One study followed children who had been undernourished at the age of three. When they were examined at age 11, it was found that, on average, their I.Q. (intelligence quotient) was 15.3 points lower than the average for their age group.30

Deficiencies of three specific nutrients are globally recognized as causes of lowered mental health among children: iron, iodine and protein. In most Western countries, it is believed that the problem of iodine has been properly dealt with by the addition of potassium iodide to table salt. This has certainly been successful in preventing goiter, the most overt sign of iodine deficiency; however, the opinion of some outside-of-the-windmill doctors today is that there is a wide gap between prevention of goiter and whole-body iodine sufficiency. We will dedicate a few lines to this subject in a later chapter.

Lack of iron has been connected to poor brain development and to cognitive problems, in addition to the physical weakness of anemia. Children deficient in iron have been found to be nervous and restless and, therefore, they create disturbances in the classroom. When trying to diagnose a child's behavioral problems, this problem should be added to the checklist (before drugging the kid). One generally-accepted-for-no-good-reason-as-far-as-I-can-tell practice may be a cause of low iron in babies: clamping the umbilical cord immediately after birth. When this is done, the newborn does not receive his God-intended amount of blood with its iron (and oxygen). I suggest that all pregnant woman request that the umbilical cord be allowed to pump for at least three minutes after birth, a request generally granted by doctors and midwives.

---

29 *Relationship between hunger and psychosocial functioning in low income American children.* J.M. Murphy, et al. Journal of American Academic Child Adolescence Psychiatry, 37(2): 163 70. 1998.
30 *Malnutrition at age 3 years and lower cognitive ability at age 11 years: independence from psychosocial adversity.* J. Liu et al. Archives of Pediatrics and Adolescent Medicine, 157(6): 593-600. 2003.

Low protein consumption, when it exists, is usually found among economically weak populations. In this case, the problem is not one of knowledge (the kind of problem I hope this book will help resolve), but of financial means. For a solution to this type of problem, we must depend on governmental and private organizations, and on the good hearts of individuals. The problem of feeding people with adequate protein could be called "the malnutrition of the poor."

We will occupy ourselves with the other kind of malnutrition, "the malnutrition of the rich." Is such a thing possible? Don Quixote's **"Yeessss!!!"** echoes back to us from the other end of the canyon. The malnutrition of the rich stems from our straying from natural nutrition. Strangely, the most blatant sign of this type of malnutrition is excess weight, even obesity! Yes, obesity is the result of malnutrition! When the food we eat is deficient in even one of the elements vital to health, the switch that shuts off the desire to eat does not drop. Empty calories, those unaccompanied by nutrients, do not satisfy. Excess sugar turns into body fat, excess fat in the food also becomes body fat, and despite the fat accumulating in the body, the child continues to eat.

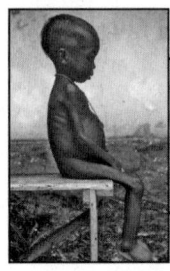
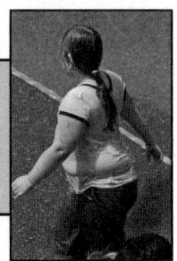

THE TWO FACES of MALNUTRITION

Weight problems — too much or too little — are not the whole story of malnutrition, of course. We can say that the great majority of children in all countries are damaged by malnutrition to some extent, if we delve deeply into the subject and define the concept broadly:

Photos: (left), U.S. Government, Centers for Disease Control and Prevention; (right) Walter Siegmund, 2007.

MALNUTRITION: *A condition whereby, due to a deficiency in one or more nutrients, an individual does not achieve the optimal physical and/or mental—emotional—spiritual condition, which he would achieve if the deficiency did not exist.*

Using this definition, we cannot always discern whether a person suffers from malnutrition. It is possible for a young man or woman to be as strong as an oak tree, as beautiful as the dawn, successful in everything, and yet not quite fulfill some exquisite potential due to a minor lack of some nutrients needed for the proper functioning of a few of the thousands of biochemical reactions necessary for optimal physical or mental functioning. Because of the wondrous uniqueness of each soul, science will never be able to achieve the exacting knowledge necessary to actually diagnose or treat such a situation. So, what should we do? We live in an imperfect world, and we accept this fact. Paraphrasing the words of a Talmudic sage: "The work is great. We can never complete it, yet we can not free ourselves from the obligation to try." It is certainly the obligation of every parent to strive continually to provide their children with quality food, and to distance them from harmful foods and environmental influences — to strive to live according to the 14 rules outlined in Chapter 1.

Another important contribution to solving the problem of nutritional deficiency is knowing about and using nutritional supplements: vitamins, minerals and others. Conventional doctors are very rigorous about requiring high level proof of efficacy and safety before recommending the use of any supplement, but generally their caution is wildly exaggerated or totally unfounded. The public, on the other hand, does not need to prove, but to decide. We are free to swallow a supplement because "It makes me feel better," or "It helped my aunt," or "It makes sense, I believe in it," or "I read in the newspaper about an experiment which shows that…." All these are not accurate evaluations, certainly not enough for a scientist, who needs large, random, double-blind, controlled trials (comparing a test group to a group that received a placebo — a sugar pill), written up in an important medical journal. If these trials have not been conducted and published, the tendency among doctors is to relate to "Not proven to be safe and helpful" as "Proven *not* to be safe and helpful." There is a vast difference between these two concepts.

This care taken by doctors before recommending any supplemental nutrient seems, on the surface, praiseworthy, since it fulfills a major medical principle: "First, do no harm." What's this I hear??? Yes, it's Don Quixote: **"Wiiindmilllls!!! Chaaaarge!!!,"** he commands. What kind of incredibly gigantic double standard is at play here!!! If only the extreme caution in following this rule was directed towards prescription drugs! Many of them have been found to be damaging or even lethal, if not immediately, then after years of mass public use. Yet, they are handed out by the billions every day.

"If we doctors threw all our medicines into the sea, it would be that much better for our patients and that much worse for the fishes."
— Oliver Wendell Holmes, M.D.

The anti-inflammatory drug, Vioxx, is thought by many to have killed tens of thousands of people by heart attack before its use was restricted. Estrogen replacement therapy, originally thought to be the Fountain of Feminine Youth, sentenced countless women to death by cancer. Many drugs have been pulled off the market after causing great damage and, in some cases, it has been found that the companies producing them hid negative studies which would have prevented introduction of the drug into the market.

Apparently, most people assume that the benefits of a drug far outweigh the risks, or else the authorities would not permit its use. We, the students of Don Quixote, however, have our doubts. Do you think that all of the evil people work for cigarette companies, while the righteous work for pharmaceutical companies? Nope. Same mentality. The existence and profitability of cigarette companies **prove** that commercial interests **can** cause people to **intentionally** override their human decency and sell something that kills people.

Many believe that cigarette advertising is **intentionally** designed to subliminally draw our young people into a lifelong addiction to cigarettes. Many believe that drug company executives **intentionally** create markets for poisonous drugs which are marketed as disease-treating substances, while in truth they only treat symptoms.

The most profitable drug does not cure a person, yet can be sold to him for decades. Do you think that a pharmaceutical windmill is interested in curing heart disease? Can you imagine them creating a pill which, after the first bottle, is not needed because the person is cured? Very bad for business. Remember, a pharmaceutical company is just like a company that sells cigarettes or brooms or chocolate or cars: the primary goal and obligation is to make profits to return to investors and shareholders. The pharmaceutical industry includes companies which are among the most profitable in the world. User, beware. As Owen Fonorow, moderator of the Vitamin C Foundation forum and author of the book, *Practicing Medicine Without a License*[31], likes to say: "Doctors learn everything they think they know from drug companies."

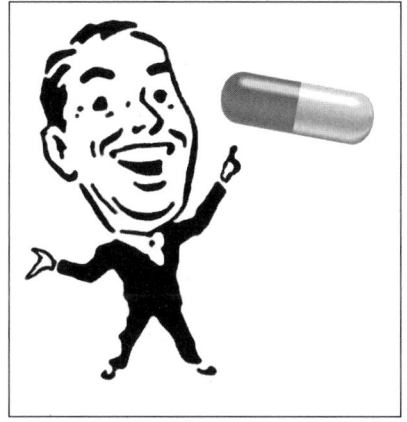

In truth, there really is justification for not using the same standards of risk management when evaluating drugs and most nutritional supplements. However, the windmill world has it all backwards. *Prescription drugs* should be controlled *much* more strictly, and far more leniency used in recommending nutritional supplements as medicine. Any decision to offer a substance for treatment should consider the benefit-to-risk ratio. It is inherent in the definition of a patented prescription drug that the molecule used is foreign to the human body. Therefore, the body does not "know" enough about

---

31   Fonorow, Owen. *Practicing Medicine Without a License?: The Story of the Linus Pauling Therapy for Heart Disease.*2008. Available from *www.lulu.com*.

how to use it, regulate it, break it down and excrete it. A natural molecule cannot be patented. You can not patent air, water, vitamin D or magnesium. If a substance cannot be patented, it is of no interest to a drug company. The fact that anyone can sell it creates competition, which prevents raking in absolutely obscene profits. Nor is there any motivation to support expensive research proving that such a substance is useful in preventing or curing disease. That is the simple reason why vitamins are not officially "proven" to be curative, a fact used as a weapon against them. (Even here, I must add that there truly is an insurmountable amount of evidence for the great benefits of vitamin treatment; however, being detrimental to windmill interests, this is criminally denied and ignored.)

A patented medicine is foreign to the human body. It is designed to block or strengthen a natural biochemical process, usually an enzymatic pathway. The aspiration of drug developers is to create a "magic bullet" which will hit only its target, without causing collateral damage. This goal has never been reached, because any chemical material that enters the body participates in many processes, not in just one. This is one of the miracles of Nature, the Efficient. A very limited number of natural nutrients are necessary to build the body and help it function, perhaps less than fifty. Many different cell types have receptors for the same molecule, which has varied effects in the cells. Admitting a foreign substance like a prescription drug into the bloodstream is like throwing a wrench into a gearbox. You never know in advance what damage will be caused. Because of the great biochemical individuality that exists in each of us, we can never be sure that a drug will not cause severe negative reactions in a small portion of the target population, sooner or later.

According to official sources, drugs may be causing the death of more than 100,000 Americans each year, even when they are used correctly![32] (You are hereby invited to compare this number to the number of people who were killed in the Twin Towers attacks,

32   Lazarou J, Pomeranz B, Corey P. Incidence of adverse drug reactions in hospitalized patients. JAMA. 1998;279:1200-1205.

a one-time event which shook the foundations of the United States. Where is the outrage about medicine-death?!?!) Millions more each year suffer from side-effects, and many more die from mistakes made by doctors and nurses when administering drugs. Despite all this, pharmaceutical drugs are used, because the benefit-to-risk ratio is assumed to be positive.

Take out your thesaurus for this one. In stark, blatant, clear, obvious, manifest, palpable, conspicuous and transparent contrast to the above, no one dies from taking vitamins. Their negative side effects are rare and mild, contrary to headlines in the media scattered about by windmills worried about their "healing" monopoly. We, meaning humanity, have about 70 years of experience taking large and small doses of vitamins and minerals in the form of supplementation. If they were truly dangerous, we would surely know about it by now. I would like to direct a simple question to those who proclaim the dangers of these substances, the first question a detective asks upon arriving at a crime scene (I actually saw this on television): "Where are the bodies?"

Of course, there are some contraindications for taking certain supplements in certain situations, and so a certain amount of knowledge is necessary, but compared to taking prescription drugs, the dangers of nutritional supplements, in general, are like a peashooter compared to a modern tank. When a substance is not dangerous, and research and/or clinical observation and/or personal experience and/or scientific rationale indicate that there may be some benefit from the substance, then one can be very lenient about the demand for absolute proof of benefit before recommending its use.

This is the case when recommending a multivitamin/mineral supplement (we'll call it a multi, for short). Since we can assume that we have nutritional deficiencies even though we eat "correctly," it would seem logical and wise to take a supplement containing small quantities of as many nutrients as possible. The multi answers this need. It is similar to a food, since food, too, has a wide variety of nutrients. In fact, since a good multi is a package of nutrients with few or no calories, we may say that it is the most nutrient-dense food available. Rather than seeing the multi as medicine, a concept that has some negative connotations attached, it is fitting to consider it a food, something a healthy person eats, too. What can parents do in a real world with real nutritional problems? Start by giving your child a multi. It's good for the body and good for the soul, and only costs a few dimes a day.

The general conclusion from research is that even slight malnutrition influences a child's I.Q.[33] At least 15 studies were conducted, examining the influence of a multi formula on various measures of children's learning ability and behavior. The results were mostly positive, especially in tests measuring non-verbal learning, short-term memory and visual perception, all of which are expressions of processes taking place in the more ancient parts of the brain. As expected, the level of improvement associated with taking the multi was greater in parallel to the severity of the baseline nutritional deficiency of the children examined.[34]

Interesting research was also conducted as to the effect of a multi on violent behavior among children. In one project, a multi, containing only 50% of the recommended daily allowance (RDA) of each nutrient (considered *very* minimal amounts by Don Quixote's students), was given to a group of forty children, aged 6 to 12, every day for four months. As a comparison, a second group of forty children was given a fake supplement (a placebo). The experiment was double-blinded.[35] The end-point of the experiment was the comparison of the number of cases in which disciplinary measures

33   *Influence of malnutrition on intellectual development.* Upadhyay SK, Agarwal DK, Agarwal KN. Indian J Med Res. 1989 Dec;90:430-41. PMID: 2628311

34   *Micro-nutrient supplementation and the intelligence of children.* Benton, D. Neurosci Biobehav Rev. 2001 Jun;25(4):297-309. PMID: 11445136

35   To isolate the results from psychological influences, no one in either the test group or the placebo group knew whether they were receiving the real pill or the placebo, made from inactive ingredients. This is the first "blind." The second "blind" was that the people who were actually giving the pills to the children and recording the results, and therefore were relating to them personally, also did not know which type of pill each child was receiving. In this way, their possible influence on the participating children, and the possible unintentional skewing of results were eliminated. Only the trial designers, who had no direct contact with the participants, knew who was receiving what.

had to be taken due to anti-social behavior. Indeed, during the study period, discipline was needed only on the average of once per child in the group of children receiving the active pill, compared to 1.875 times in the control group, an improvement of 47%. Eight types of behavior were recorded: threats/fighting, vandalism, defiance, obscenities, refusal to work or serve, endangering others, and various offences. In the words of the study's authors:

> CONCLUSION: Poor nutritional habits in children, that lead to low concentrations of water-soluble vitamins in blood, impair brain function and subsequently cause violence and other serious antisocial behavior. Correction of nutrient intake, either through a well-balanced diet or low-dose vitamin-mineral supplementation, corrects the low concentrations of vitamins in blood, improves brain function and subsequently lowers institutional violence and antisocial behavior by almost half...[36]

In this chapter, we have primarily discussed minor nutritional deficiencies, and how they cause behavioral and learning problems in children. In Part II, we will consider the nutritional basis for more serious diseases and disturbances.

Well, since we spent a lot of time researching the benefits of breakfast, let's dedicate a short chapter to the subject. What can we give our children for breakfast in order to minimize the possibility of our dear ones being damaged, body and soul, by the malnutrition of the rich or of the poor? And, if you please, how do we get them to eat the good eats? That's a tough subject, but we'll try.

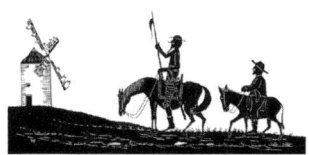

36   *The effect of vitamin-mineral supplementation on juvenile delinquency among American schoolchildren: a randomized, double-blind placebo-controlled trial.* Schoenthaler SJ, Bier ID J Altern Complement Med. 2000 Feb;6(1):7-17 Department of Sociology and Criminal Justice, California State University PMID: 10706231

Chapter 4

Breakfast

"My child does not want to eat 'healthy'!"

You are right, dear mother or father. All the philosophies are worthless, if your child will not eat what is placed in front of him. And so, I will express myself with all of the tact which I have gathered unto myself through the years: *the problem is not the child.* The *parent* often believes that children only like sweet junk foods. The *parent* often is afraid even to suggest a better way. A number of times, I was surprised to see with what ease a child accepted menu changes. Did I just make you laugh? Perhaps your child is of the other variety: screaming, kicking, complaints, refusal… No big deal, proceed slowly. Speak to your child's heart, just as you would speak to an adult. Explain in terms the child understands — this good food or supplement is brain food. Every child understands that a brain is a good thing. Or, "Good food makes your skin prettier," which works best on budding teenagers. Use your hard-earned wisdom to know what motivates your child.

It is usually unnecessary to assert authority, which can create opposition in even the smallest child. There are better ways. Speak to your children of nature, of how the earth provides our food, of how plants gather sunlight and use chlorophyll to turn light into energy. Speak to them of the blessings of water, cycling from clouds to earth, to plants, to us, to the drainage system, to the oceans and back to the clouds. God, or Nature, gave water to the beasts and birds and insects to drink. Are there cola ponds in the jungle? Show them the amazing pictures of water crystals from the work of Masaru Emoto.[37] Share the earth with your children, dig it and fertilize it with compost, even if only in a pot on the windowsill. Show them the natural compost on the forest floor. Plant a seed and let them nourish it. Speak to them of nature's colors, point out the bright red of a tomato and the orange of a carrot — colors that make miracles in our bodies. Speak to them of the purity and holiness of their bodies and souls, deserving of the blessings of good food.

Our youngest son happily eats whole grains with tofu and, of his own initiative, he adds flax oil. He doesn't like white spaghetti, because it has no taste; he prefers his spaghetti brown. I watched my daughter's son, at the age of one and a half years, eat pomegranate seeds with gusto, and another little grandson cry until he was given another "little tree" of cauliflower. Be creative and "educate the child according to his way"[38]. And the main thing: be a good example.

Speak to them of junk food, too. Show them the falsehood of advertising, and how the creators of colored boxes don't care about what happens to the children who eat the stuff inside. Explain that the stupid two-cent toy inside is given not because of love, but only to get a child to whine at his mother until she buys the whole box. One face is worth a thousand words, so practice puckering in the mirror, while saying "Yuck!" Pucker your face in distaste when you tell your children about false food colors, preservatives, empty calories and cigarettes. Show them pictures of black lungs and breathing tubes. Speak to them of knights and windmills, about valor and bravery, of seagulls that flew beyond the flock. Talk to them about

---

37   Emoto, M. *The Hidden Messages in Water, The Healing Power of Water* and other books. *The Secret of Water* is written for children. Emoto used a special photographic technique to capture the shapes of frozen water crystals. He found that when water was exposed to prayer, beautiful music and even a word — such as "Love" — taped on the container, the crystal was very beautiful. When the water was exposed to something negative, the shapes were likewise negative.
38   *Proverbs* 22:6.

lemmings, about individuality, about the strength to be unique and not follow the stupid herd.

As a first, unavoidable step to healthy breakfasts, throw out the sweetened breakfast cereals. (I don't recommend giving them to your cat or dog, because they also need real food.) Besides all the sugars and artificial chemicals in these products, the grains on which they are based have been debased, subjected to processing that has destroyed their nutritional value almost entirely: soaking in chemical baths, cooking at high heat, smashing and puffing. In short, their nutritional quality is almost nil. In fact, I once read about an experiment in which a group of mice was fed water and puffed wheat, while another group was given only water. You'll never guess who died faster. Please do not fall prey to claims printed on cartons about the wonderful health qualities of the products enclosed and how they are enriched with vitamins and calcium. This is like a thief who strips his victim bare and then has mercy and gives him two dollars for a bus. (By the way, what is the difference between adding vitamins to breakfast cereal and taking vitamins in a capsule? Why does the former merit praise from the windmill organizations, while the latter is generally dismissed as unnecessary? Could it be, as Don Quixote has hinted, that one is good for the food industry and the other is not?)

Parents buy the ease of serving packaged cereals: box, plate, milk, spoon... job finished. No need for creativity and no complaints from the little ones. Children are sold on the colorful cartons, become addicted to the sugars and manufactured tastes, and then suffer their whole lives from mental and physical weakness, and finally disease and degeneration, the true products of the food industry. If your child really gives you a hard time, well, it won't hurt him one bit to miss breakfast once or twice because there is no junk in the house. Parents, just be strong. *When all is said and done, there is a reason that God made the world in such a way, that parents are big, and children are small.*

Breakfast Ideas

(These are in no particular order. The list is intended to provide easy solutions that will not take more than a few minutes to prepare.)

- ❤ *Oatmeal.* My momma used to serve me hot oatmeal with a pad of butter and some brown sugar melting on top, their colors swirling in the milk and the smell wafting up my nostrils. Instant oatmeal is probably not as good as the cooked variety, which takes only a few minutes and has that old down-home feeling. Oatmeal is an excellent breakfast food, which releases its nutrition for hours. Kids relate to it like dry cereal. (Sneak in a bit of extra brown sugar if you need to. I won't tell Don Q.) Make sure that the oatmeal you buy is whole grain and not refined. Oatmeal is best cooked in a pot, but if time is short, boiled water can be poured directly over the oats in the bowl, especially if they are finely ground.

- ❤ *Other whole grain, cooked cereals*: amaranth, barley (not pearl barley, which has had too much of the brain removed), buckwheat (kasha), cornmeal, millet, rye, quinoa, rice. These are excellent foods for any meal. As is true of oatmeal, they provide steady energy for hours. Take care when you read product labels, and make sure the product provides true whole grain nourishment. We must learn to be discerning consumers, as some terms can be misleading:

  - ✦ "Made with whole grain" means that there is *some* whole grain in it, but not *only* whole grain. You may notice that the ingredients say, "Flour, whole wheat flour...." The first and most weighty ingredient is refined flour.

  - ✦ "100% wheat" means "but not 100% *of* the wheat kernels."

  - ✦ "Multigrain" means more than one grain, not that any of them are whole.

+ "Stone ground" sounds good, and quite possibly the grains ground are whole, but not necessarily. The phrase only refers to the grinding process.

♥ *Whole grain breads*, toasted or not, with butter, cheese, avocado, jam (without sugar or chemical preservatives) or other creative spreads. (Note: pumpernickel always looks like whole grain, but is not unless marked as such.)

♥ *Eggs*: one or two, scrambled, soft boiled, hard boiled, poached, or whatever else one does with eggs. Contrary to some opinions, eggs are an excellent food for most people, as long as there is no allergic reaction. Eggs are a whole protein, meaning that all the essential amino acids are present. In fact, eggs are the standard against which other protein foods are compared. There is no need to worry about cholesterol. The "cholesterol causes heart disease" thing will someday be broadly recognized as the nonsensical fraud it is. It is one of those nutritional "facts" which are barren of fact.

♥ *Granola or muesli.* (Read the labels and watch out for highly-sugared products.)

♥ *Fruit*:

+ *Shakes*: cut almost any fruit combinations and toss them into the blender for a few seconds. When bananas get overripe, rather than throwing them out, freeze them and use them as part of the shake. A bit of milk, yogurt or water makes the shake more liquid. Apple juice concentrate, maple syrup, honey or stevia (a sweet herb which comes in powdered or liquid form) will make the shake sweeter, if necessary. Almonds or ground flax seed, tossed into the blender with the fruit, thicken the texture and enrich the brew. Be creative and make a delicious, nutritious breakfast for your children.

+ *Fruit salad*, with or without yogurt.

✦ *Juice.* Any fruits or combinations; add some vitamin C powder, if you can (regular ascorbic acid powder is sour, which imposes a limitation on the amount added. Use it as you would use a lemon).

❤ *Pancakes or waffles* from whole grain flour. Sweeten with honey, stevia or maple syrup.

If after all, you must keep a box of commercial cereal in the house for emergency situations, such as if you have 30 seconds to get out of the house and you need to put something in a plastic cup for the kid to take, carefully select a cereal with the least number of ingredients whose names you can't pronounce, and the least amount of sugars. You can sweeten simple bran flakes, for example, with honey, maple syrup or jam made from 100% fruit.

Chapter 5

FNOBC
(Faulty Nutrition of Brain Cells)

Old Medical Truth:
You cannot make a diagnosis if you don't think of it.

The brain of a child is like a crystal, collecting light and color, pictures, sounds and words, smells, tastes and physical stimulation through the sense organs, skin and nervous systems, which transfer their impressions of the outside world through nerve fibers to the brain. The brain processes all this input using its amazing and singular abilities, and, in the end, it shines forth something totally new to the world. The number of brain cells is like the number of stars in the heavens; but rather than being surrounded by a vacuum, they are surrounded by a liquid environment of thousands of different types of molecules for their nutrition.

A large body of scientific literature has been developing the idea that optimal concentrations of key nutritional molecules are not always provided by our food. A deficiency in one or more of these molecules, or of the atoms which form them, may adversely affect optimal brain function, and may be expressed as mental and/ or emotional disturbances — soul disturbances — including ADD (Attention Deficit Disorder), hyperactivity or more serious mental diseases. The last seventy years has seen the development of a medical approach called orthomolecular medicine ("ortho" = correct or fixing), in other words, using the correct molecules to heal. These molecules are usually natural to the human body, as opposed to patented medicines, which are basically poisons taken at a non-lethal dosage, intended, hopefully, to bring about healing. The goal of the orthomolecular approach is to deliver optimal concentrations of nutrients to the cells of the body, thus treating health problems at the source. If cells are healthy, then the tissues that they build will be healthy. If tissues are healthy, then the organs built from them will be healthy. If organs are healthy, then their owners — you, me and our children — will be healthy.

The use of patented medicines has been called *toximolecular medicine* by practitioners of orthomolecular medicine, because the molecules of pharmaceutical medicines are toxic at doses not far above therapeutic doses. The practitioners of toximolecular medicine have not called orthomolecular medicine anything. They prefer to ignore orthomolecular, nutritional medicine, denying its existence with flimsy denials and a wave of their hands, as though the authoritative letters "M.D." were a magic wand. Actually, we students of Don Quixote, believers in the orthomolecular approach, are sometimes called quacks. And what do we say to that? "Quack, quack" is what we say, as we continue to help people heal.

FNOBC: Faulty Nutrition of Brain Cells

This diagnostic label was invented by yours truly, as a general term describing the basis of much of what is called 'mental illness', an expression that doesn't tell us much at all.

A diagnosis is meaningless if it does not point to a possible treatment. So, is this diagnosis, "faulty nutrition of the brain cells," a real, workable diagnosis? Your doctor will never tell you it is, because the term does not appear in medical school textbooks. Your psychiatrist also will never make this diagnosis, because it does not appear in his bible, the DSM (Diagnostic and Statistical Manual of Mental Disorders). The pharmaceutical companies *certainly* will not tell you about this diagnosis, because it appears not in their accounting books and will never contribute to The Bottom Line. But in my book, the answer is, "Yes, this is a real diagnosis, and a very practical one." It is very general, of course, since the "faulty" part covers a wide variety of possible faults. However, when these faults are recognized and clarified, the path of treatment is often clear and the results powerful. The expression of these faults varies from person to person over a wide range, beginning with nervousness and lack of inner peace, through hyperactivity and attention deficit disorders, depression and outbursts of anger, to any and all of the serious psychiatric disorders, of the kinds listed in the bible of the psychiatrists.

Now let's discuss some of the major types of faulty nutrition of the brain cells — hereby called FNOBC — which can affect the soul of your child, and how to avoid them, recognize them and treat them. (I was going to call it FNBC, but it sounded too much like it could be a TV network. While we're on the subject of TV, staring at one, or watching the wrong programs, causes a different type of faulty brain nutrition. In fact, certain shows cause immediate mind rot.)

Excess consumption of simple sugars

Possibly the first practitioner of modern medicine to treat psychiatric problems with nutrition was Dr. Abram Hoffer (1917-2009), a Canadian psychiatrist and biochemical researcher. In the 1930's, an experiment was done in which a group of mice was given a low-calorie diet. The distance these mice ran around in their cages was measured and compared to the distance run by well-fed mice. The well-fed mice ran three miles in a day, while the underfed mice ran seven miles, as if restless, perhaps searching for food. A couple of decades later, Dr. Hoffer repeated this experiment with one difference. The mice receiving the restricted diet were given the same number of calories as the control group, but their diet was lacking in the B group of vitamins. Guess what? The same results were seen! As the low-vitamin group ran and ran and ran, Dr. Hoffer realized that the mice were *hyperactive!* Dr. Hoffer began treating psychiatric problems from hyperactivity to schizophrenia with vitamins, laying the foundations of "orthomolecular psychiatry," an advanced, evidence-based method of psychiatry that seeks to supply brain cells with their proper nutritional environment. This system directly treats the *roots,* not only the symptoms, of psychiatric problems,: faulty nutrition of the brain cells. The phrase "orthomolecular" was coined and applied to Hoffer's work by the most famous chemist of the last century, Linus Pauling, who was awarded two Nobel prizes and is considered "the Einstein of chemistry."

The process by which most cellular energy is created is called the Krebs cycle, a series of chemical reactions which give off ATP, the "currency" of cellular energy, produced when glucose[39] is "burned." Certain vitamins and minerals must be present in order for the Krebs cycle to proceed. If you *ever* wondered what typifies all the B vitamins, and why they are grouped together and called "B complex" (and this is true even if you never wondered about it at all), well, the answer is: all of them are involved in the Krebs cycle. Without any one of them, the cycle would not turn, and energy would not be produced. These vitamins are essential for life.

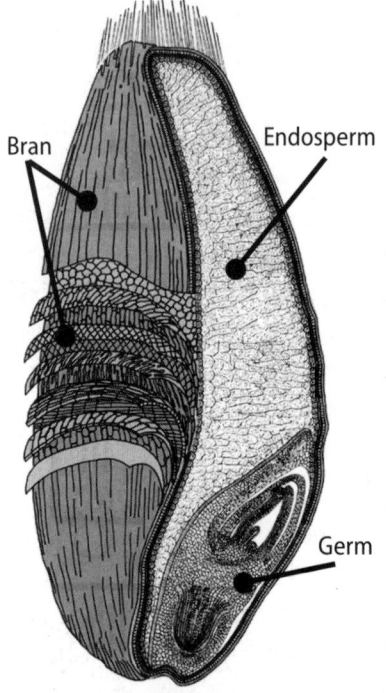

Bran

Endosperm

Germ

Courtesy of the Wheat Foods Council

The wheat seed, from which flour is ground, is made up of starch (endosperm), bran and the germ. Starch is

---

39   Glucose is the most important sugar. It is formed from other sugars, as well as from fats and amino acids which form proteins. White sugar, sucrose, is made of one molecule each of glucose and fructose.

nothing more than bunches of branched glucose chains. White flour consists of starch only, the germ and bran having been removed. Nature created the seed in a wondrous manner, so that whoever eats the whole seed consumes, in the bran and the germ, the exact vitamins and minerals needed to produce energy from the starch. When we, the wisest creatures on the face of Earth, remove the bran and germ to make our lovely, white flour, from whence does the Krebs cycle gather the vitamins and minerals necessary to produce energy? From the stores already existing in the body, of course. In this way, deficiencies of these nutrients are created. Therefore, anyone regularly consuming products made from white flour and white sugar is guaranteeing himself the development of critical nutritional deficiencies, damaging his body and brain, and causing FNOBC. This is why white sugar has been nicknamed "the white thief," a name equally deserved by white flour.

Understanding the root of a health problem makes it easier to find an effective treatment. A deeper look into the Krebs cycle reveals which nutritional factors lead to the kind of FNOBC caused by consuming simple sugars. The rule here is: every nutrient involved in producing energy from sugar, but not consumed along with the sugar, is suspected of causing FNOBC and its resulting problems of the soul. While it is unnecessary to get lost in the complexities and details of the Krebs cycle, a brief glance at the drawing on the right will deliver the message of the importance of B vitamins in the cycle. The circled acronyms refer to molecular compounds containing a B vitamin. Clearly, B vitamins are involved in almost every step.

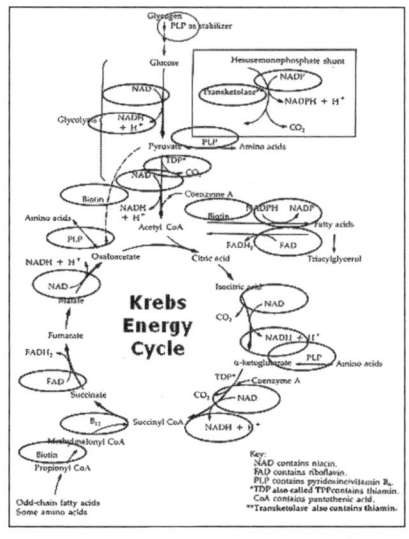

Several minerals also have a part in the Krebs cycle. It is interesting that these same minerals are also found in the parts of the wheat kernel removed in the process of manufacturing white flour and in the parts of sugar cane or beets removed when white sugar is purified. These include magnesium and chromium, necessary for the peace of your child's soul in many ways. The parts removed are also dietary sources of fiber, important for digestion and the health of the digestive tract.

Another major category of public damage caused by food industry companies, the modern windmills, by their intentional temptation and entrapment of the public into addiction to simple sugars, is:

Reactive hypoglycemia, the imbalance of blood sugar levels

Eating simple carbohydrates — white flour products and sugar — causes a sharp rise in the concentration of sugar in the blood and the corresponding excretion by the pancreas of insulin, whose job is to push sugar into the cells. When the rise of sugar in the blood is too fast, the resulting insulin blast drives sugar out of the blood too quickly and overshoots, dropping the blood sugar level too low. Since a steady and continual supply of glucose to the brain is necessary to life, an alarm is sent to the adrenal glands, and they release stress hormones designed to raise the blood sugar level to proper balance. This is part of the famous "fight or flight" response, since our muscles need elevated sugar levels to provide energy for fighting or fleeing.

The adrenal hormones stimulate emotional stress and physical nervousness, resulting in outbursts of anger ("I could kill for chocolate!") and other intense reactions. As the level of sugar *must* be raised, an uncontrollable desire for carbohydrates rises as the body takes over control from the mind. Sugar is eaten, and the cycle repeats. This vicious cycle is called "reactive hypoglycemia," expressing itself as addiction to eating simple carbohydrates, unstable emotions, vitamin and mineral deficiencies, and exhaustion of the adrenal glands, leaving the sugar-addict physically exhausted and unable to respond to the normal stresses of life. The end result of this process is often diabetes.

Children are especially sensitive to this type of hypoglycemia. In one study, adults and children drank water containing glucose. Their glucose levels were measured at various intervals to see if there is a difference in how adults and children process elevated sugar levels. Both groups' sugar levels rose and then fell almost identically; however, their responses to the reactive hypoglycemia were very different. The children's adrenalin levels rose more than twice as high as the adults', showing that the reactive hypoglycemic cycle is particularly vicious among children. Researchers concluded that reactive hypoglycemia and its resultant adrenalin rush "may be important contributing factors to adverse behavioral and cognitive effects after sugar ingestion [even] in healthy children."[40] What wonderful love we give children when we reward them with sweets! What great birthday parties we make for them!

Treatment options for FNOBC
caused by simple sugar consumption

The above technical explanations lead to one conclusion related to the treatment of children with suspected FNOBC or to its prevention: **take action in every way possible to limit your family's intake of simple sugars!!!** (Please take a moment to contemplate the significance of the three (3) exclamation marks, which Don Quixote asked me to insert).

Removing simple sugars from your daily menu and embarking on a new path is a major part of treatment; however, a regimen of nutritional supplements must also be considered to treat the deficiencies caused by your old diet. When digging a hole, stopping the dig will not fill the hole. Moreover, if you have ever dug a hole and then tried to refill it, you may have noticed that the dirt you took out no longer

---

40   Jones et. al, *Enhanced adrenomedullary response and increased susceptibility to neuroglycopenia: mechanisms underlying the adverse effects of sugar ingestion in healthy children.* Department of Pediatrics, Yale University School of Medicine. J. Pedeatr. 1995. PMID:7844661.

fills the hole completely; more must be brought from somewhere else. Similarly, the "hole" in nutrient satiety caused by faulty nutrition needs more than just an improved menu. Usually, "megadoses" of some nutrients are required, or, as the doctors who developed the orthomolecular approach say, "optimal doses." Why is the amount of vitamin C needed to cure a cold called a "megadose"? Why is the amount of vitamin E used to prevent diabetic neuropathy called a "megadose"? A teaspoon of vitamin C is called a megadose, but the same amount of sugar, the raw material from which most mammals manufacture vitamin C in their livers, is added to millions of cups of coffee daily without a second thought. It would be more fitting to call a teaspoon of an unhealthy substance like sugar, which can *cause* a person to catch a cold, a megadose, and to call the amount of the substance that can *cure* that same cold an "optimal" dose.

In the case of sugar-induced FNOBC, which can contribute to ADHD or worse, a child should be given an adult B complex supplement containing 50 milligrams of each of the main B vitamins. There are also multivitamins containing this amount of the B complex vitamins, along with RDA amounts of many other vitamins and minerals. This is excellent, since faulty nutrition must have also caused at least minor deficiencies in many other nutrients. In some cases, extra-large doses of vitamin B3 and/or vitamin B6 are necessary; this, however, requires the diagnosis and guidance of a knowledgeable therapist. In later chapters, more will be said about these vitamins.

Taking supplements has another advantage, making it possible to be a bit less strict in making necessary dietary changes. It is not a good idea to embark on a radical dietary program which will cause your child to feel deprived. In such a situation, she may be driven to eat sugar whenever away from parental supervision. Your child will get the message and cooperate if you explain the reasons for the changes. Help her consider herself a partner in a mission, in taking on a challenge. Some research has shown that if a reasonable amount of sugar is included in a balanced meal, hyperactivity will not result. Dr. Conners, of the Psychiatric Department of the Children's

Hospital in Washington, found that sugar consumed with protein and starch does not cause immediate problematic behavior. We, the true students of Don Quixote, look upon research of this type with a suspicious and critical eye. Furthermore, even if problematic behavior is not *immediately* evident, nutritional deficiency will progress nonetheless. In any case, we live in the real world and are ready for some compromise (just a little bit) when the hard-earned wisdom of life calls for it. Please do not tell D.Q. on me for saying that.

Smooth and Easy

One of the most important minerals for human health is magnesium. There are 140 milligrams of magnesium in 100 grams of whole wheat flour, but only about 25 milligrams in white flour. In molasses, produced from the initial pressing of sugar cane, there are 150 milligrams of magnesium in every 100 grams, whereas white sugar has none. Therefore, a child fed a diet high in simple sugars will most certainly develop a magnesium deficiency, which exists in the majority of our modern population and causes untold and unrecognized suffering. Magnesium is the mineral of "smooth flowing," a calming influence on both physically and mentally. Magnesium deficiency is characterized by the *lack* of smooth flow, as evident in constipation, high blood pressure, muscle cramps, premenstrual syndrome, nervousness, emotional instability, sleep disturbances and hyperactivity. Indeed, magnesium deficiency is a form of FNOBC that contributes to *every* disturbance of the soul. Magnesium participates in at least three hundred enzymatic reactions, so a deficiency of this mineral has broad repercussions. Since it is often difficult to diagnose magnesium deficiency by evaluating symptoms, and blood tests do not give an accurate picture of magnesium status in cells and tissues, it is wise to assure proper intake.

General improvements in nutrition should slowly raise magnesium levels; however, taking specific measures should be considered. Foods rich in magnesium include nuts and seeds, bulgur (wheat groats) and buckwheat, carob powder, blackstrap molasses and green leaves. (In the center of the chlorophyll molecule — the green color in plants — sits an atom of magnesium, just as in the hemoglobin molecule — which gives the red color to blood — sits an atom of iron). There are also various forms of magnesium supplements. A recommended dry form is magnesium citrate, found in some commercial supplements, although the majority contain the cheaper and less absorbable magnesium carbonate. Magnesium chloride — crystals, liquid or oil — is an excellent form, especially for children, as it can be massaged on the child's back or belly — adding the important parental touch "nutrient" — or added to bathwater, as the magnesium is absorbed well through the skin. I have seen children with asthma helped by magnesium chloride. Maybe it was the mineral only, but a parental back rub may also be considered an important part of the treatment protocol. Love heals!

Astronaut!

A vitamin B12 deficiency can develop for several reasons. Parents of vegetarian children, especially those eating a vegan diet (total abstention from animal products) must be especially diligent, since most of our B12 consumption is from animal products. It is not certain that these children will develop a deficiency, since vitamin B12 is manufactured for us by "good" bacteria in the intestines. Children taking antibiotics regularly, however, can not rely on this source, because antibiotics kill beneficial bacteria along with harmful ones. Some vegetarian foods contain some B12: fermented soy products (miso, soy sauce, natto and tempe), seaweed and algae. Since some experts, for various reasons, are uncertain about the efficiency of these sources in supplying the necessary amounts of B12, caution is always recommended.

The clearest signal to check your child's B12 level is if he is lightheaded or, for lovers of classical English, "spaced out." While this condition can be caused by other things, it may be a warning sign of B12 deficiency, which can lead to anemia and damage to the nervous system. Even children who eat meat can develop a B12 deficiency. The absorption of this vitamin is very complex, and various digestive problems can impair its absorption.

Treating B12 deficiency

Whenever a child has a problem with concentration, even if ADHD has not been diagnosed, his vitamin B12 blood level must be checked. If a deficiency shows up, treatment is very simple: a daily dose of B12 in an amount dependent on the child's size and the recommendation of a knowledgeable person, or a weekly shot until the level normalizes. Once the body's storage of the vitamin is full, it should suffice for at least a half year, even if the child's diet is less than optimal. If B12 deficiency is causing problems of attention and concentration, there is nothing stupider ("or more evil," says Don Quixote) than giving a child a drug rather than B12, and yet this probably happens every day. A child with a Ritalin deficiency has yet to be found!

Imbalanced fat intake

Much of the weight of brain tissue is composed of essential fatty acids (essential fats). As our body chemistry does not manufacture them, we must receive them from food. There are two families of essential fats: omega-3 and omega-6. For the purpose of our discussion, we are usually speaking about inadequate consumption of omega-3 fats. One of these, DHA, is one of the most important materials in the brain, found mostly in brain cell membranes. DHA is highly unsaturated, making it very liquid. This makes it ideal for active cells like brain cells, which continuously change shape, reaching out with arm and leg-like projections to make new contacts with neighboring cells. This is sometimes called plasticity, and is vital to thinking, learning and memory. Lack of DHA, which is replaced by fatty acids of less efficient function, is an important form of FNOBC. A large body of research points to the influence of omega-3 intake on various mental and emotional states and learning ability: depression, bipolar disorder, dyslexia[41] and ADHD[42]. Omega-3 intake during pregnancy may influence your child's I.Q. years later. DHA is so important for the development of the fetus' central nervous system[43], that it will "rob" this material from its mother. If a mother does not have enough for herself as well as her baby, she will end up with a deficiency, possibly the main cause of post-partum depression. Every pregnant woman should take an omega-3 fish oil supplement.

The need for attention to omega-3 is the result of a basic imbalance existing in our modern diet between different types of essential fats. The general population nowadays receives omega-6 from many foods, whereas omega-3 has almost disappeared from our food chain. The healthy omega-6 to omega-3 ratio is estimated to be from 1:1 up to 4:1, as it was in the diets of earlier societies. Today, the ratio in our diets may be 20:1 or greater. This imbalance, a form of FNOBC, has several combined causes:

- Our meat comes from cows raised on grain mixtures completely lacking in omega-3, rather than from animals eating pasture grass, which has omega-3.
- The same for our eggs.
- Fish are the major source of omega-3 today; however, fish truly rich in omega-3 are found only in cold ocean waters, where liquid fatty acids are needed to avoid sluggishness of cell membranes. Fish raised in pools are doubtful sources. We also tend to overcook fish, which destroys omega-3.
- The consumption of oils from seeds and beans: soy, corn, sesame. All these are high in omega-6 compared to omega-3.
- The consumption of margarine, which is high in omega-6

41   Stordy BJ. *Dark adaptation, motor skills, DHA and dyslexia.* Am J Clin Nutr 2000 Jan;71. PMID 10987373.

42   Burgess, John et al. *Long-chain PUFA in children with ADHD.* Am J Clinical Nutrition, Jan 2000. PMID: 10617991

43   Innis SM. *The role of dietary n-6 and n-3 fatty acids in the developing brain.* Dev Neurosci 2000 Sep-Dec;22(5-6):474-80. PMID 11111165.

and unnatural fatty acids. In the past, there was no such thing as margarine; instead, butter was made from milk from pastured cows, and animal fat was used for frying.

- The consumption of baked goods containing hydrogenated and partially-hydrogenated oils. These are damaging to health, since processing changes the natural shape and structure of fatty acids. "Trans fats," and other unusual forms of fat, are formed. These replace essential fatty acids in biological systems and disrupt the functioning of these systems.

In addition to problems of the soul, fatty acid deficiency symptoms include vision impairment, high triglycerides, eczema, dry skin, edema (swelling caused by fluid retention), tingling sensations in the arms and legs, weakness and tissue inflammation.

Treatment of essential fatty acid FNOBC

Since the causes of omega-3 deficiency FNOBC are clear, the treatment also becomes clear:

- Reduce consumption of the foods listed above that contain only omega-6, along with trans-fats and other unnatural creations. Olive oil can replace commercial soy, corn and sesame oils most of the time.
- Eat fish containing omega-3: tuna, salmon, sardines, anchovies and herring. There are some problems hidden in this rule, as some of these fish may not be from cold oceans, but from fish farms in other places. There is also growing concern about the dangerous presence of mercury in fish. Therefore, it is not a good idea to eat a lot of fish. Measures must be taken to prevent and clear out the collection of mercury in our bodies — a subject we will deal with later on.
- Eat walnuts and pumpkin seeds (less important sources, but sources nonetheless)
- Omega-3 is found wherever there is chlorophyll, so dark

green, leafy plants contain omega-3. Wild plants are especially healthy.

- Use organic eggs. Some egg boxes indicate that the eggs are rich in omega-3, which means the hens either grazed on grasses or ate flaxseed.

- Use seaweed and algae: spirulina, chlorella, kombu and others. These have been used to revive populations suffering from severe malnutrition, such as the survivors of the concentration camps after the Holocaust. The omega-3 in these foods helped renew brain function.[44]

- Supplements: Supplementing omega-3 intake is among the most basic and important treatments of children suffering from ADHD and most of the other disorders discussed in this book. Choosing a proper product for children takes some effort. Most products for adults contain capsules the size of a small torpedo, so not all children are willing or able to swallow them. If they can, they should, as the dose for an adult is good for a child also. There are many omega-3 products designed for children, in liquid form or small capsules. The dosage must be examined. In addition to DHA, there is another important omega-3 fatty acid called EPA. Whereas DHA plays a mainly structural role, EPA is involved the communication between the membrane and the genetic material in the cell's nucleus. Most supplements have a combination of EPA and DHA. To evaluate a supplement, simply add the amounts of EPA and DHA together. The minimal dose for an ADHD child is a total of 300 milligrams of these two fatty acids combined. There may also be a figure for "total omega-3", or "total fish oil", which you can ignore. It usually is unnecessary to spend your money for extra essential fatty acids of the omega-6 or omega-9 (from olive oil) variety. You and your child most likely get a

---

44   Pitchford, Paul. *Healing with Whole Foods*. 1993, North Atlantic Books. pp. 122-125.

sufficient amount of these in your diets to make the amount in the supplement negligible. Simply add up the EPA and DHA, and ignore the rest. We recommend a capsule form rather than a liquid, since liquid forms need all sorts of other ingredients, often including sweeteners, to cover up omega-3's fishy taste; however, if your child has difficulty swallowing capsules, liquid is a solution. A child with ADHD should *always* be given an omega-3 supplement.

- Use flaxseed and flax oil. Flax seeds can be purchased in most health food stores; some types are golden and some are brown. They should be whole and in good condition. Grind a week's supply in a coffee grinder and keep it in the freezer. The amount of omega-3, in the form of ALA (alpha-linolenic acid), can be as much as 25% of the weight of the seed, making flaxseed the richest source of omega-3 in the plant kingdom (at least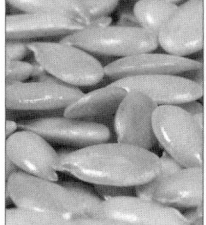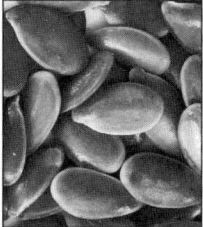

Flaxseed

on dry land. In the oceans, ALA-containing algae and plankton are the source of omega-3 for fish). Flaxseed oil is also available, fresh (maximum 3-4 months from pressing), refrigerated and in a dark bottle. Fresh flax oil has a light, pleasant taste. If it tastes bad, it is spoiled.

It must be noted that the omega-3 fatty acids found in flax seeds and other vegetable matter is not the same as the omega-3 from fish or animal products. This ALA must undergo conversion (elongation and desaturation) in the body to form the active omega-3 fatty acids, EPA and DHA. Some people may have problems making this conversion, such as deficiencies of required enzymes; therefore, it

Photo credits: (light flax seed) en:User:Bdevel [Wikipedia]; (dark flax seed) Sanjay Acharya is more therapeutically efficient to obtain omega-3 from fish and other animal products, or from supplements. The fish have already done the work for us of converting plant omega-3 to its active forms.

As a rule, the forms of omega-3 can be compared thus: two tablespoons of flaxseed = one tablespoon of flax oil = approximately 600 mg of EPA + DHA, although there is a wide range of estimates of this final figure. The different estimates, in truth, might all be correct in different people, depending on how well their bodies make the conversion. In addition to their omega-3 content, flax seeds have other inherent health benefits. Mahatma Gandhi said: "Wherever flax seed becomes a regular food item among the people, there will be better health."

Flax seed: How to Use — How Not to Use
- Sprinkle on salads, grain and bean dishes.
- Mix with oatmeal, yogurt or applesauce.
- Use in soups — pour into the soup bowl, not the cooking pot!
- Do not use flax oil or seed in frying — the hot temperature changes the oils into toxins.
- Baking: do not use flaxseed oil to oil the pan, nor the seeds to sprinkle on top, because the surface temperature is too high. Mixed into the dough, however, the seed is protected from air, light and heat. The inside of baked bread is actually steamed at an acceptable temperature.
- Since flax seed absorbs five times its weight in liquid, make sure to drink adequate liquid.

Iron
Most of the body's iron is used to make hemoglobin, where it sits in the center of this large molecule. It also is contained in the myoglobin molecule in muscle. Both these molecules supply oxygen to the cells, and so the proper amount of iron is vital to human function. Although enough iron is usually obtained from food, deficiency is not

uncommon, and can cause symptoms similar to those of ADHD. Iron deficiency is a cause of anemia, the symptoms of which are shortness of breath, weakness, fatigue, heart palpitations and a sore tongue. Deficiency in infants and young children is associated with slow mental development and learning difficulties. Iron is best absorbed from animal sources. Vitamin C is known to aid iron absorption.

On the other hand, too much iron can cause a child to be aggressive, over-emotional and hyperactive, and is considered a strong risk factor for heart disease later in life. Therefore, supplemental iron should only be given when blood tests show that iron is lacking. Keep iron supplement bottles out of the reach of children, as there have been cases of overdose and even death when children took too many iron pills at once. The causes of deficient levels of iron are complicated, and even Don Quixote agrees that conventional medicine knows how to diagnose and treat iron problems. Our role here is to awaken awareness that a child with ADHD or other problems may have iron excess or, more likely, a deficiency. If so, he does not need ~~Speed~~ Ritalin.

This chapter has covered the major relatively common, relatively easily noticed, and relatively easily treated nutritional deficiencies affecting the soul of the child. There are many other nutrient deficiencies, but most of them are filled by general dietary improvement, without giving special attention to eating foods rich in the particular nutrient and/or taking it as a supplement. If a person eats a whole-food diet which attempts to mimic as best as possible the foods of primitive cultures, he will come closer to healthy nutrition, especially if his diet is supplemented by a multivitamin/mineral supplement. Using other specific supplements according to the orthomolecular approach is a vital and important branch of nutrition and *medicine*, and expert advice from an orthomolecular practitioner is recommended for treatment of any health disorder. Many other conditions can cause forms of FNOBC, such as digestive problems which impair absorption, infection which uses up nutrients, ingestion of medicines which cause nutritional deficiencies, environmental toxins which use up antioxidants and can block the actions of nutritional minerals, and health conditions which raise the need for some nutrients. We will discuss many of these subjects in later chapters.

Get used to the word,
"orthomolecular"!
It's the medicine of the future!

Chapter 6

Vitamin "L"

LOVE changes body chemistry, as well as affecting the obvious: the soul of the child.

Part of what defines a vitamin is that it must come from an outside source, because not enough of it, if any, is manufactured in the body. In this respect, LOVE really *is* a vitamin. Life is impossible without every single vitamin. I guess you could say that, technically, life can carry on without LOVE, but I'm sure you agree, that life without LOVE could hardly be called living.

Home cooking does not destroy vitamin L; in fact, by a process not yet quite explained by modern scientific methodology, vitamin L enters food straight from loving hearts in the kitchen. Much of this vitamin is lost when food is refined. Although there is *some* vitamin L in the junk food passed out at birthday parties or given as a replacement for proper hugging, the form of vitamin L in these foods is mutant, and apparently blocks the receptor sites for the real thing.

Love is seeing the best in your children. You are not here to belittle them and tell them they are not good enough. The rest of the world will try to teach them this lesson. They need you to believe in them, so that they will believe in themselves. This kind of vitamin L actually improves their I.Q. In an eye-opening study[45] in

---

45   Rosenthal and Jacobson. *Teachers' expectancies: determinants of pupils' IQ gains.* Psychol Rep. 1966. Aug;19(1):115-8. PMID: 5942071

1966, an intelligence test was given to all the pupils in a San Francisco elementary school. The teachers were told that certain children in each class showed unusual potential for intellectual gains. Eight months later, these "unusual" children showed significantly greater improvements in I.Q. than did the others. *These children, however, had actually been chosen randomly, the only difference being the teachers' expectations!*

According to laws of spiritual magnetism understood throughout the ages, your thoughts and expectations affect your children. Dream for your children and help them dream for themselves. Accept them with unconditional love for who they are. Your children are spiritual beings sent to be your guides, as well as to be guided by you. Your hearts are the best nourishment you can give to them, and they will gift you plenty of Vitamin "L" in return. Dance to your baby's crib when her crying wakes you up at night, for this is a heavenly privilege.

I learned a wonderful lesson one day a couple of decades ago. My wife was in the hospital on pregnancy watch with our fifth child and the other four were at home, making a mess for me to clean up. Picture me, with a "why me" attitude, carrying two heavy baskets of groceries from the local store with the rain pouring on my head. Suddenly, a light turned on inside me, and I realized, "Hey, it's all BLESSINGS!!! — a wife to worry about — a new soul on the way — four beautiful children at home — a real home — baskets full of food — the world needs rain... BLESSINGS AREN'T EASY! *And,* I have enough strength to carry it all!"

Accept your blessings and bless others. Especially, bless your children, and give them plenty... of LOVE.[46]

---

46 My thanks to Elson Haas, M.D. and Buck Levin, Ph.D., R.D., in whose excellent and recommended nutrition textbook, *"Staying Healthy With Nutrition"* (2006), I first encountered the term "Vitamin L." My apologies to the Japanese research group led by Dr. W. Nakahara, who used the expression "vitamin L" to describe factors reported to be essential for lactation in rats, and proposed to be necessary for proper human metabolism. Vitamin L has also been used as a nickname for the mineral lithium. Neither the lactation factor nor lithium are proven to be essential for humans, so they are not proven to be vitamins. LOVE, therefore, wins the title.

*"...I will act, says Don Quixote, as if the world were what I
would have it to be, as if the ideal were real..."*
— Don Quixote de la Mancha, Cervantes

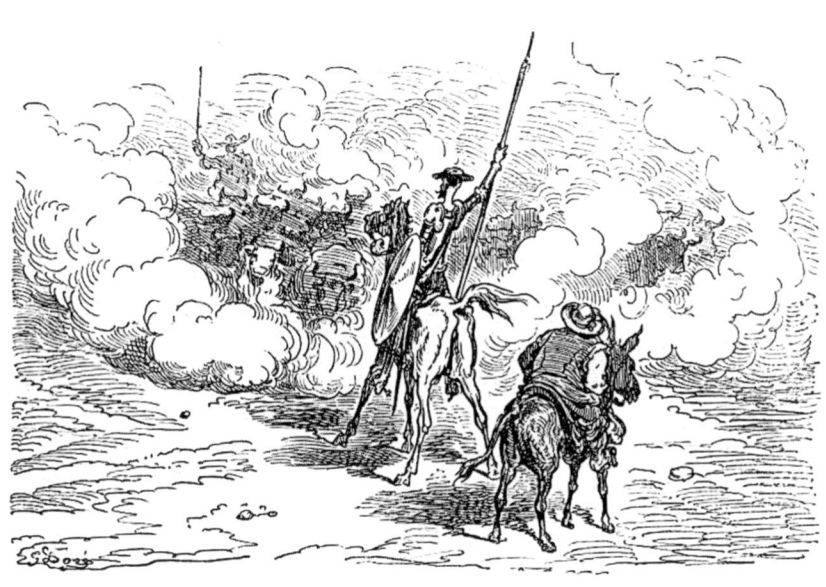

Chapter 7

In the Beginning:
Pregnancy, Birth and Nursing

"And God created man in His own image... male and female He created them. And God blessed them; and God saw every thing that He had made, and, behold, it was very good."

Mother, do you know when proper nutrition for your child started? No, not when you got pregnant or just before that. It started when you were in *your* mother's womb. By the time you were born, you had a couple million itsy bitsy eggs in two baskets — your ovaries. These eggs were "Survival" applicants, and the winner turned out to be the egg from which your child would someday "hatch."

Remember the difference between organic and inorganic eggs from the first chapter? So, you see, the nutritional power in that winning egg depended on what *your* mother ate! The other half of the material from which your child was created — a mighty sperm — won a swimming contest against 200 million competitors, racing blindly but fearlessly down a dark tunnel, slamming full speed into the victory prize, fertilizing the egg! Your child is a born winner!!!

It's a good thing that, in your mother's time, the quality of food was better, properly nourishing the original you, and the eggs inside you. There's not much you can do about your early nutrition. No amount of past-life regression therapy can change the nutrition *you* received before you were born, but you *can* help your descendants from now on. Starting right now, your job is to provide proper nutrition for your born and unborn children — and for your grandchildren inside *them*.

The development of your child's soul is greatly influenced by what you eat and how you take care of yourself before and during pregnancy, and when you nurse your baby. I urge you to do everything you can to enter pregnancy without bad habits, health problems or nutritional deficiencies. Improper preparation could mean a difficult pregnancy and years of recovery for you, as well as affecting your child's health and learning abilities. The child's father must also take care of himself, as nutritionally healthy men provide smarter sperm. During pregnancy, the body needs more of everything — calories, protein, vitamins and minerals, as well as both rest *and* activity. It takes about 75,000 calories to make a baby, or about 350-400 calories a day, so mothers-in-waiting must eat 20-25% more than usual. These calories should come from nutrient-dense, quality food.

Dr. Weston Price, our hero and nutrition guru from Chapter 1, wrote at length about nutrition and pregnancy. Dr. Price's explanation of this illustration teaches us some awesome lessons:

> The oldest child, ten years of age, is shown at the upper left. She has a marked underdevelopment of the width of the face and dental arches. The nostrils are abnormally narrow and she tends to be a mouth breather. She is very nervous and is becoming stooped. In the lower left photograph is shown an x-ray of her narrowed upper arch. At the right is shown her younger sister, six years of age. It will be seen that the proportions of her face are much more normal and that she breathes with complete ease through her nose. She has none of the nervous trouble of her older sister. In the x-rays below, at the right, it will be seen that her permanent arch, as indicated by the positions of the permanent teeth, has good design.

> The history of these pregnancies is of interest. The duration

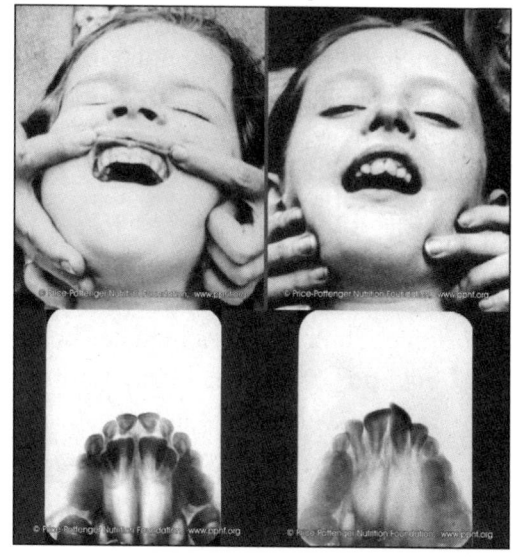

of labor for the first child was 53 hours and for the second three hours. Following the birth of the first child, the mother was a partial invalid for several months. Following that of the second child the experience of childbirth made but slight impression on the strength and health of the mother. During the first pregnancy no special effort was made to reinforce the nutrition of the mother. **During the second pregnancy the selection of foods was made on the basis of nutrition of the successful primitives.** [Emphasis added.] This included the use of milk, green vegetables, sea foods, organs of animals and the reinforcement of the fat-soluble vitamins by very high vitamin butter and high vitamin natural cod liver oil.[47]

A couple of comments are in order about the selection of foods. The quality of most of these foods today is lower, so nutritional supplements are necessary, as explained below. In addition, we cannot recommend cod liver oil, because the vitamin A content of this oil is too high and can cause birth defects if too much is taken.

Since we are not living in traditional tribal societies or isolated mountain villages, we have new nutritional concerns, beyond improving our food's quality. Several supplements are vital to support the pregnant mother and her baby. Here are most important of these, along with other tips and important information:

---

47   Price, Weston. *Nutrition and Physical Degeneration*, pp 405 and 408.

- **A prenatal multivitamin:** Every brand of this type of multi gives small amounts of many nutrients, adjusted for the minimal needs of the typical pregnant woman. Consider this a very nutrient-dense type of food. The multi should be started at least a month before pregnancy.
- **Folic acid** is found in every prenatal multivitamin, but it is mentioned here on its own because of its importance, and because it *must* be taken if, for any reason, you do not want to take a prenatal multi. It has been clearly shown that folic acid prevents spina bifida (Latin for "split spine"), a birth defect involving the incomplete closure of the embryonic neural tube. It is less known that this closure happens very early in a pregnancy, before many women even know they are pregnant, and so a mother must have a proper folic acid level even before conception. Folic acid is found in green, leafy vegetables, dried peas and lentils and in supplements. The minimum dose is 400 mcg daily, and up to 1,000 mcg can be taken without medical guidance. Although this is one of the few nutrient supplements whose benefits are wholeheartedly accepted by institutional medicine, even today not every pregnant woman takes folic acid. Do it!
- **Vitamin C** is a basic foundation of health, with benefits too numerous to mention here. None of the fears about vitamin C, implanted in your brain by uninformed ignorant sources or by informed malevolent sources, has any basis. The only limitations on vitamin C intake are imposed by your bowels. If you take more than you actually need, your bowels will loosen, a harmless side-effect which informs you that you can be confidant you have taken enough of this vital nutrient until tomorrow. Dr. Frederick Klenner was a pioneer in the vitamin C arena for several decades, beginning in the 1940's. At his North Carolina hospital, the babies born to mothers under his care were called "Klenner babies" by the nurses, because of their robust health. Klenner gave

pregnant women 5,000 milligrams of vitamin C daily in the first trimester, 10,000 in the second semester and 15,000 in the third. If that sounds too incredible or undoable, you can at least take 3,000 milligrams a day, dividing it into three doses — morning, noon, and night — MINIMUM. *Your doctor will try to scare you out of your vitamin C. Nod your head up and down, say "Uh huh" and then ignore her.* Note that this is one of the few places in this book that I am explicitly suggesting that you ignore your doctor. I'm that sure about this. **The only contraindications to taking more than two grams a day are if you have familial hemochromatosis (genetically high iron levels in the blood) or G6PD deficiency (a genetic lack of this specific enzyme), or if you are one of those rare people whose bowels will audibly beg for mercy at the minimum suggested level.**

- **Iron**: Since blood volume rises in pregnancy by 50%, you need 50% more iron in your diet. This may come from red meat, chicken, salmon, seaweed, brewer's yeast, molasses, spinach, chard, nuts, seeds and legumes. However, it is difficult to get enough iron without a supplement. Prenatal multivitamins contain iron.

- **Omega-3**: An omega-3 fish oil supplement should be taken by every pregnant woman, right along with her vitamin C and prenatal multi, which does not contain omega-3. For more details, review the chapters on FNOBC and ADHD. I will just remind you here that without enough omega-3, a pregnant woman risks post-partum depression and seeing her child suffer from learning disabilities in school, years later.

- **Vitamin D**: A low level of vitamin D at the beginning of pregnancy increases the chance of preeclampsia (see below) by five times, even when taking 200 or 400 I.U. in a prenatal multi. Check your 25(OH)D blood level before getting pregnant, and take at least 2,000-5,000 I.U. daily until you have reached the minimal healthy level of 50 ng/ml. Although this level of intake is perfectly safe, you may have to educate your doctor about this, too. Full body, "unprotected" sunning is also an effective way of raising your vitamin D level, and is safe, *as long as you avoid getting a sunburn*. The dangers of sun exposure have been exaggerated; sunblock blocks vitamin D production in the skin, exposing us to the many serious dangers of vitamin D deficiency. Vitamin D is actually a hormone that acts on at least 200 different genes, which means that it has at least 200 ways of acting on the human body.

- **Iodine**: if any of your thyroid hormone levels are low, as evidenced by a TSH test, or if you have symptoms of hypothyroidism — unexplained weight gain and tiredness, feeling cold, thinning hair, "fog brain" — it is vital for you and your baby that you supplement iodine. This is true even if your TSH is within the range, but near the upper limit. (More on this in Chapter 12, "The Good.") Sufficient iodine is important for you *and* your child's soul.
- Replace regular sodium-chloride table salt with high-quality sea salt containing no aluminum silicate or other material to make it "flow". Aluminum is suspected of contributing to autism and causing Alzheimer's disease, so a lifetime of flowing salt consumption is inadvisable. Sea salt is a natural, whole food containing many helpful minerals. Dr. Price included salt in a short list of foods consumed and valued in *all* native cultures. Don't overdo it, but use it.
- Avoid all drugs — legal or illegal — including caffeine (sleep if you are tired), artificial sweeteners and other unnatural food additives. Medicines should be taken only when absolutely necessary. Do **not** get dental amalgams put into your mouth during pregnancy.
- Do **not** get a flu shot during pregnancy! While the mercury-

containing substance, thimerosal, has been removed from most vaccines since the beginning of this century, in 2002, the Center for Disease Control began recommending flu shots for pregnant women[48], a practice not approved even by the FDA. Most flu shots contain mercury, which doses up the fetus! The wise CDC also recommends these shots for infants from 6 to 23 months of age, restoring up to 60% of the thimerosal dose which had been voluntarily removed. This is probably a reason that removing mercury from most vaccines does not seem to have reduced the incidence of autism, a subject discussed in later chapters. If you take enough vitamin C, your chances of getting the flu drop off the charts.

- Preeclampsia, or toxemia occurs in about one out of every twenty pregnancies and causes tens of thousands of deaths every year. Its symptoms are high blood pressure, protein in the urine, swelling, weight gain, headaches and vision problems. If you improve your diet and take the supplements listed here, your chance of suffering from preeclampsia, gestational diabetes and other problems will be minimal.

Experience birth! (Easy enough for me — a male — to say.)

Pregnancy, birth and nursing should be a very special time, connecting you to the divine, to the source of wisdom at the depth of your being. Nature's glory is revealed. The depths of love are opened.

Many practices encouraged or performed by modern medicine, such as use of epidural anesthesia during birth, are based on our cultural avoidance of pain and struggle at all costs. Many women have allowed their conscious minds to overwhelm and block the

---

48   Bridges, et al. *Prevention and Control of Influenza — Recommendations of the ACIP*, April 12, 2002/51(RR03);1-31. *www.cdc.gov/mmwr/preview/mmwrhtml/rr5103a1. htm.* PMID:12112171. Thank you to *Medical Veritas International* for directing me to this source from their article, *www.medicalveritas.com/manGoldmanYoung2.pdf.*

feelings rising from their souls, the internalized Word of God, so to speak, embodying the first commandment in the Garden of Eden: "Be fruitful and multiply." The act of birthing should be filled with internal joy. Yes, birthing is usually very painful, but women who are properly prepared and have the proper attitude understand that it is a good pain, gifting the new mother with feelings of victory and empowerment, and an increased bond to her child. We have been conditioned to avoid pain and struggle, to take painkillers for every headache and physical pain, however minor. We have been taught to take antidepressants to dull soul pain. If you have a headache, take a pill and keep working. If your marriage is difficult, get another one. If your child is different, drug him.

If you fear childbirth and ask your doctor for an epidural, you are missing something. You may also be doing some violence to your baby. The drug you get, your baby gets, albeit to a lesser degree, as the placental barrier filters out some of the drug. The following describes the short-term effects of an epidural on newborns. (Other researchers have not seen such negative reactions and consider epidurals to be safe.)

> Significant and consistent effects of bupivacaine [the epidural drug] ... can be demonstrated. Immediately after delivery, infants with greater exposure to bupivacaine *in utero* were more likely to be cyanotic [appearing blue, due to insufficient oxygen in the blood] and unresponsive to their surroundings. Visual skills and alertness decreased significantly with increases in the cord blood concentration of bupivacaine, particularly on the first day of life but also throughout the next six weeks. Adverse effects of bupivacaine levels on the infant's motor organization, his ability to control his own state of consciousness and his physiological response to stress were also observed.[49]

The long-term effects are unknown. It *may* be reasonable to as-

---

49   Rosenblatt, et al. *The influence of maternal analgesia on neonatal behavior: epidural Bupivacaine.* International Journal of Obstetrics and Gynecology, 1980. PubMed: 7225300

sume that there are no serious long-term effects on a child's learning abilities, but we don't know for certain in every case. Since our love is greater than our need for scientific proof, we worry about effects that are so mild as to be unnoticeable and unprovable. As usual, biochemical individuality is a major problem when using any drug millions of times. Even a small percentage of sensitive individuals becomes significant, even if the overall benefit/risk ratio is good. For this reason, when the major reason for using an epidural is merely pain avoidance, drug avoidance should take priority.

A woman given an epidural, essentially paralyzing the lower half of her body, becomes detached from that is happening and cannot participate in the birth. Labor time is increased and all kinds of things happen. Who do you want to be in charge of your birth process, Mother Nature or a doctor?

While studying about epidurals, I read complex medical discussions about when, how, where, dosage, supporting drugs, dealing with side effects and more. Why should it be so complicated?!?! Is birthing something that humankind has to figure out a better way of doing? Maybe Mother Nature has birthing worked out already; intervention into her ways had better have a good reason. Of course, doctors should be involved in the birth process. However, they should be there to watch over, not replace, natural birthing, ready to use their knowledge and experience in an emergency. Sometimes, there are good reasons to administer an epidural, but not usually. Epidurals should *not* be routine.

Transfusion

Another questionable practice… Actually we should say what we believe — another senseless, damaging and criminal intervention into Mother Nature's ways is the routine clamping of the umbilical cord immediately after birth, interrupting the natural infusion of blood into the baby. Are we smarter than nature? Do all mammals on earth have defective blood-infusion systems for their newborns? Can we possibly be correct in deciding that the blood supply that babies receive right after birth is excessive?

In the minutes after your newborn comes into the world, her body transforms from being an organ of her mother — on the delivery route of blood from her mother's heart — to independence. Suddenly, within a few minutes, her own internal systems must do everything. Suddenly, oxygen must come from her own lungs into her own blood supply. That famous, awaited first cry is our sign that she is alive on her own. Her own blood must be plentiful, rich in nutrients, and under enough pressure to flow into the farthest reaches of her circulatory system, flooding the vessels of her brain, for each cell must feast or die. Blood floods her liver and her kidneys, and these begin their lifelong job of filtering and purifying blood. A myriad of changes take place, intricately timed and connected, designed to support her life for a hundred and twenty years. All this must happen within five minutes, because after just five minutes, the umbilical cord becomes still, the pumping of blood through it is over, the transfusion of the vital fluid is finished, and your baby is on her own. *But she NEEDS this five minutes to get her BLOOD SUPPLY, and who do you think you are, Doctor, clamping it off after less than a minute!!! Are you smarter than GOD???*

Okay, okay, even Don Quixote was shocked by my outburst. But I've been reviewing this stuff and writing about it for the last several hours, and I feel sick to my stomach thinking about the damage and suffering this cord clamping might have caused already, and about how, while I write, it is being done to still more babies!

Clamp the cord to prevent neonatal jaundice, you say, Doctor? This condition is almost always benign and goes away by itself. No proof that clamping causes damage, you say? The burden of proof is on *you*. Go ahead, prove it by a controlled study. Do placebo cord clampings!

When the cord is clamped, immediate asphyxia is produced: the baby gets no oxygen until her lungs function. If this does not happen within six minutes, even doctors know that permanent brain damage will result. Oxygen is our most vital and urgent nutrient. Why do doctors demand proof that minor brain damage does not occur after only two or three minutes, causing subtle, untraceable behavioral or learning defects that will not show up for years? How can they possibly require *proof* of harm to convince them to stop clamping off a baby's blood supply? Clamping robs a new human of up to half her birthright blood. She could have iron deficiency anemia, which may result in language and motor disability, sometimes irreversible. Anemia is thought to be the primary cause of these disabilities. It's not. Cord clamping is! And if it is, the treatment of anemia has limited success. Some researchers believe that cord clamping is the major cause of the increase of autism. Move over mercury, you have competition!

Prove it, you say, Doc? Prove it's *not*, I say.

Another thing very injurious to the child, is the tying and cutting of the navel string too soon; which should always be left till the child has not only repeatedly breathed but till all pulsation in the cord ceases. As otherwise the child is much weaker than it ought to be, a portion of the blood being left in the placenta, which ought to have been in the child.
— Erasmus Darwin, Zoonomia, 1801

See, even Charles Darwin's grandfather agrees with me!

Nursing and the soul of the child

Oxytocin is wonderful. This is the feel good, "shower the people you love with love"[50], generosity and bonding hormone. It is created in the body by the vaginal stimulation of childbirth labor and by the kind of love that began the process nine months earlier. At that time, the bond was deepened between the baby's father and mother. Oxytocin encourages and shortens labor. (An epidural administered during labor lowers a mother's oxytocin blood level[51]. It is certainly

---

50   The title of a song written by James Taylor, as most of you probably know.
51   Rahm, et al. Acta Obstetricia et Gynecologica Scandinavica, *Plasma oxytocin levels in women during labor with or without epidural analgesia: a prospective study.* Vol. 81, Issue 11 November 2002. PMID: 12421171.

at least one of the ways an epidural prolongs labor, in addition to detaching a mother from her physical and emotional connection to her lower half.) After birth, stimulation of her nipple during nursing causes a mother's body to produce oxytocin, which passes from her blood into her breast milk, and then into her baby's blood.[52] Aided by oxytocin, the bond between mother and baby is deepened at this time, as both souls are deeply nourished.

Nutritionally, no man-made formula can ever truly replace mothers' milk. We can make a formula by adding one isolated ingredient to another and then another, while breast milk contains myriads of substances, many of which we have not even identified. Breast milk contains living white blood cells and antibodies from the mother that will protect her newly-independent child from foreign invaders until his own immune system develops, as well as supplementary hormones, digestive enzymes and essential fatty acids, such as DHA, which is difficult to put into manufactured formulas because it spoils quickly. The vitamins and minerals in breast milk are in molecular forms perfectly designed for human babies. Breast milk contains more vitamin L than any formula ever could. Breast-feeding nurses the soul of the child.

What science says about breast milk vs. formulas:

- A Danish study tested the intelligence of over 3,000 men and women of the average age of 27, and found that "Duration of breastfeeding was associated with significantly higher scores on the Verbal, Performance, and Full Scale IQ tests."[53]
- Breastfeeding has been shown to be associated with a reduced risk of obesity in later life.[54]

---

52   Takeda et al. *Concentrations and origin of oxytocin in breast milk.* Endocrinol Jpn. 1986. PMID 3582266.
53   Mortensen, et al. *The association between duration of breastfeeding and adult intelligence.* JAMA 2002 May 8;287(18):2365-71. PMID:11988057.
54   PMID: 16902325

- Breast milk provides better antioxidant power than formulas.[55]
- The blood of breast-fed babies kills bacteria more efficiently than the blood of formula-fed babies.[56]
- The incidence of three illnesses — lower respiratory infections, middle ear infections (otitis media) and gastrointestinal illness — was compared between 1,000 infants who were only breast-fed for at least the first three months of life and 1,000 formula-fed infants. In the first year of life, there were 2,033 excess office visits, 212 excess days of hospitalization, and 609 excess prescriptions for these three illnesses among the formula-fed infants.[57]
- Formulas cost between $700 and $3,000 a year. (That's not exactly science, but it certainly is a practical consideration.)
- People who were breast-fed as infants rise higher on occupational and social ladders, according to an English study.[58]
- Parents of breast-fed children are less likely to express concern about learning abilities, and the children are less likely to have required treatment for behavioral, conduct or mental health problems.[59]
- At the age of 10, children who breast-fed have larger lung volume.[60] Easier breathing is health-promoting. This may

55   Aycecek. *Breast milk provides better antioxidant power than does formula.* Nutrition. 2006 Jun;22(6):616-9. Epub 2006 Apr 25. PMID:16635660
56   Barriga, et al. *Serum hemolytic and bactericidal activity in breast and formula-fed infants.* PMID: 8907436.
57   Ball and Wright. *Health Care Costs of Formula-feeding in the First Year of Life.* Pediatrics Vol. 103 No. 4 April 1999, pp. 870-876.
58   Martin, et al. *Breast feeding in infancy and social mobility: 60 year follow-up of the Boyd Orr cohort.* Archives of Disease in Childhood 2007;92:317-321. Copyright © 2007 BMJ Publishing Group Ltd & Royal College of Paediatrics and Child Health
59   Knutson, Boudreau. *Breast-Fed Children Have Fewer Learning Problems,* Mental Health Diagnoses. American Public Health Association (APHA) 136th Annual Meeting: Abstract 173228. Presented October 29, 2008.
60   Ogbuanu, et al. *The effect of breastfeeding duration on lung function at age 10 years: a prospective birth cohort study.* Thorax. 2008 Nov 10. Epidemiology & Biostatistics, University of South Carolina. PMID:19001004.

also be a contributing factor to the lower incidence of asthma among breast-fed children, alongside better immune function.

- In a special online report, *The Deadly Influence of Formula in America*[61], Dr. Linda Folden Palmer has summarized the death rates among formula-fed and breast-fed infants. Averaging the findings from numerous studies in each category, Dr. Palmer concludes:
  - o Formula-fed babies have a five-fold risk of Sudden Infant Death Syndrome (SIDS). If all babies were breast-fed, over 1,500 infants would be saved from SIDS each year.
  - o About 1,200 lives are lost yearly because of heart problems and respiratory failure among formula-fed infants.
  - o If all babies were breast-fed, 300 lives every year would be saved from necrotizing enterocolitis (death of intestinal tissue).
  - o If all babies were breast-fed, 130 lives would be saved from uncontrollable diarrhea every year.
  - o The childhood cancer, neuroblastoma, strikes twice as many children who did not receive breast milk for more than one year, resulting in 20 extra deaths per year.
  - o Bacterial infection is responsible for 300 more deaths per year in formula-fed infants.
  - o Three to four deaths every year, from all causes, out of every 1,000 babies are caused by feeding them formula, rather than breast milk.

---

61   *www.naturalfamilyonline.com/articles/312-formula-report-2.htm*

We will end this chapter with Dr. Palmer's concluding words:

What Your Doctor Doesn't Tell You

Pediatricians spend much time frightening parents with something like a 1 in 100,000 combined risk from vaccine-preventable diseases when parents question the utility and safety of vaccines. "Would you want to risk the life of your child?" they demand. Yet these very same professionals offer formula samples with the other hand — when the magnitude of health risks associated with the use of formula is 500 times greater.

Parenting is all about making choices and weighing risks and benefits. Many parents need to make the riskier choice of formula feeding in order to balance other factors that benefit the family. Yet some parents who have lost their children, possibly based on pediatric advice condoning or encouraging formula-feeding, would surely wish that they had been informed of the very real risks related to using formula.

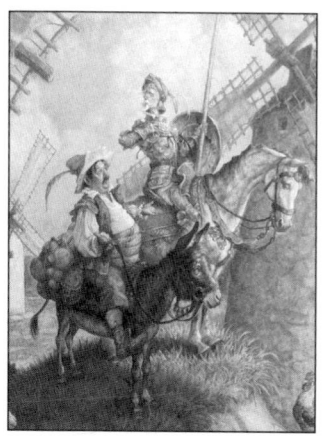

Part Two

Special Situations

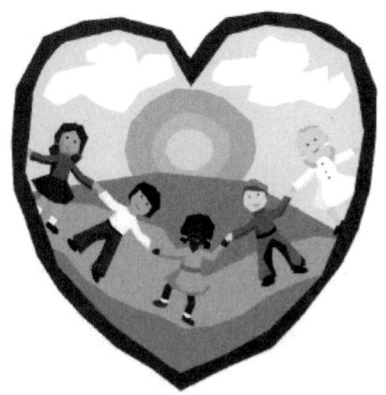

Saving One Life is Like Saving the Whole World

Step back from the bewildering world of doctors, medications and activity limitations—imagine your child living a normal life.

Chapter 8

Attention Deficit and Hyperactivity Disorder (ADHD)

The Next Albert Einstein
Sits In Fourth Grade And He's Stoned

*Early one morning, Don Quixote appeared be-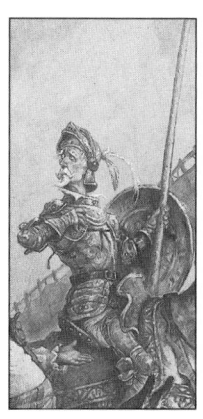
fore me, lance in hand, and yelled, "Arise, ye lazy
one!!!" "But Quixote, it's only ten in the morning!,"
I begged. "Right," said he, "I know you are used
to sleeping until noon, but millions of children
are sitting in school and they're drugged!!! Get
up and fight!!!"*

And so, here I am.

↝❧

Five to ten percent of our schoolchildren are, to some degree, drugged. Stoned, but learning. Because they're stoned, many of them have improved grades. Their teachers are satisfied, and their parents are pleased and relieved.

Attention Deficit and Hyperactivity Disorder (ADHD) is a general term, covering a variety of behavioral disorders which have worn out a series of nicknames in recent generations. In a few years, the fad will probably change and ADHD will be called something else. For the sake of style and simplicity, we will use the term ADHD for all types of attention deficit and hyperactivity disorders.

We applaud when we see children with special musical or athletic talent, but we step back in fear when we see others with certain other prominent qualities, such as a heightened need for movement, no tolerance of boredom and routine, an unusual mode of thinking or an "overdeveloped" imagination. It is impossible for children with these qualities to sit quietly in a class of thirty children and learn in the accepted way.

In our society, most of us have been conditioned, or brain-washed, to look to our medicine cabinets for solutions to all physical or emotional problems. Is it any wonder that so many children with worrisome qualities are treated with stimulant drugs such as Ritalin, antidepressants and other such "medicines," which would have numbed the creativity out of many past geniuses, denying them, and us, the fruits of their genius. We gather and wonder, we students of Don Quixote, whether these unusual qualities in children are some problem the children have, or if they are expressions of a unique and lofty destiny??? Yes, it really *is* possible that the next Albert Einstein sits stoned in fourth grade. Maybe he or she is **your** child.

I am "extra child"!

ADHD was first defined in the 1990's. It includes a variety of clinical disorders having in common various attention and behavioral disturbances. Most of these children have above-average intelligence, sensitivity and creativity. Some of them suffer from low self-esteem, due to the way society relates to their unusual behavior. As they mature, many will continue to suffer from different forms of the same symptoms, making it difficult for them to persist in the paths they choose — in school, at work, and even in marriage.

ADHD is described in *The Diagnostic and Statistics Manual of Mental Disorders* (DSM). Evaluating a child includes questioning his parents about his symptoms from early childhood, questioning his teachers, and a comprehensive physical examination that includes hearing, sight and thyroid function tests. To be awarded the title "hyperactive," or "suffers from attention deficit disorder," a child must demonstrate that he has a problem being attentive, especially in listening to details; that he makes careless mistakes, has trouble following instructions and fails to finish tasks; tries to avoid activities demanding mental concentration; is disorganized, loses things, is easily distracted and forgetful.

The problem is that this list describes "CHILD"!!!

If you were asked to describe a typical child, without using words like "small," "young" or 'short', mightn't you say that he has difficulty listening to what adults are talking about and following instructions, is disorganized and loses things, is easily distracted?

A second list of symptoms used to define hyperactivity describes a "child" even better: cannot sit still or stay in one place, runs around and gets wild, has difficulty engaging in activities requiring silence, has lots of energy, talks a lot, answers a question before it is completed, is impulsive and impatient and interrupts those around him.

So what distinguishes a hyperactive child from a normal child? **A hyperactive child is extra-child!!!**

Be objective!

How is an ADHD diagnosis made? First, as we said, the child must be extra-child. His symptoms must appear more often, be far more prominent than they are in most children of the same age, and they must continue for six months. They must influence at least two areas of his life, such as school, leisure, family time or work. The diagnosis is made according to an examiner's *subjective* evaluation. Based on their own belief systems and personal characteristics, such as patience, experience and sensitivity, different evaluators will consistently "diagnose" different percentages of children as suffering from ADHD.

When diagnosing a disease, we look for *objective* signs and symptoms. For example, when a person is diagnosed as having type II diabetes, it is clear that he has type II diabetes. There is an objective sign: the level of glucose in his blood after a 12 hour fast must be above 125 mg/dL. A doctor can get further objective data by doing an oral glucose tolerance test and by measuring hemoglobin A1C, in order to learn how long the disease has been present and how severe it is. Other symptoms are also well-defined, as is the prognosis of the disease's development.

There is, however, no objective measure of ADHD, not for the diagnosis, not for the problem's progression, and not for the results of treatment. If his teacher wakes up in a bad mood or is nervous, the child's behavior will seem, of course, more disturbing. A mother working on her doctorate is more likely to define her kids as hyperactive. From one school district to the next, different percentages of children are defined as ADHD according to totally subjective criteria, influenced by the patience of teachers and staff, the approach of the school psychologist and the parents' beliefs — their readiness to introduce their children into a process that may well lead to drug treatment, or their awareness of "holistic" concepts and natural treatment possibilities. There are no objective measures. After several people decide that a child is ill, the child will be considered ill from that moment on.

Scientific Studies

Although many attempts have been made to isolate objective anatomical or physiological differences between ADHD children and "normal" children, none have been found[62]. There have been somewhat positive-seeming results from the field of neuroimaging, in which different technologies are used to map activity in various regions of the brain. Educators and psychologists have heard of these results, and it is generally believed that objective differences have been found. This is incorrect. The major cause of excitement was a study by Giedd and his colleagues in 2001, summarizing more than thirty neuroimaging studies. "Anatomical imaging studies of individuals with ADHD consistently point to involvement of the frontal

---

62   Baumiester and Hawkins, Clin Neuropharmacol. 2001 Jan-Feb;24(1):2-10. Review. Erratum in: Clin Neuropharmacol 2001 May-Jun;24(3):180. PMID: 11290875.

lobes, basal ganglia, corpus callosum, and cerebellum."[63] In theory, if differences in brain activity are found between ADHD and normal children, neuroimaging could be used to make an objective diagnosis. However, the researchers themselves noted several limitations in the studies they examined:

1. The studies were varied, and few of the results were confirmed by additional researchers.
2. Most of the studies lacked statistical significance (meaning that the differences between the groups were so small, that there is a high possibility that further studies would have different results.)
3. The findings are "not currently of diagnostic utility."

Strengthening these doubts, in 2003, the researchers Jonathon Leo, from Western University of Health Sciences, and David Cohen, from Florida International University, published a very comprehensive article[64], reexamining the same studies analyzed by Giedd's team. They wrote:

> Giedd et al. do not provide in their tables information on …**whether or not subjects diagnosed with ADD or ADHD had a prior use of stimulant or other psychotropic medications…** information on the prior use of medication in the experimental subjects is simply too important to ignore. This is because an astronomical number of experimental and clinical studies on animals and humans find that almost every studied psychotropic drug has been consistently shown to produce subtle or gross, transient or persistent effects on the functioning and structure of the central nervous system. The very definition of "psychotropic"

---

63   Giedd, Blumenthal, Molloy, Castellanos. *Brain imaging of attention deficit/hyperactivity disorder.* Ann N Y Acad Sci. 2001 Jun;931:33-49. Review. PMID: 11462751
64   Leo, Jonathan, and Cohen, David. *Broken Brains or Flawed Studies? A Critical Review of ADHD Neuroimaging Research.* The Journal of Mind and Behavior, Volume 24, Number 1, winter 2003.

(acting on the central nervous system to produce changes in thinking, feeling, and behaving) presumes such effects.

Leo and Cohen reveal that in each and every reviewed study, either part of the test group was taking or had taken psychotropic drugs, or information on the subject was totally missing. In those studies showing a difference between ADHD children and non-ADHD children, it is probable that these differences were caused by the use of drugs, and not because of differences between the two groups of children. In other words, the data from all these neuroimaging studies do not teach us a thing! Leo and Cohen conclude:

> After twenty-five years and thirty-five studies, there is not a single straightforward experiment comparing typical unmedicated children with an ADHD diagnosis to typical controls. We are perplexed.

We, too, the students of Don Quixote, are perplexed. Be objective, dear readers, and be sure of yourselves when confronted by teachers and psychologists with a diagnosis of your child. You can rely on your knowledge that ADHD is not an objectively-defined disease or state of being. ADHD is a totally subjective diagnosis.

TOVA

One of the most popular tests used in ADHD diagnosis is the TOVA (Test of Variables of Attention). It is based on the assumption that people with ADHD have difficulty with boring, repetitive tasks. The test is similar to a computer game, where a child reacts to shapes on a screen and presses a switch. The number of times the child correctly reacts to a target or incorrectly reacts to a non-target are measured and compared to the results of peers.

While you can surely learn something about your child through this test, it does not give a "yes or no" diagnosis about ADHD. The problem is that TOVA is often used to compare a child's performance when he is under the influence of the drug Ritalin (take it easy, Don, we'll deal with this later), and when he is not. If the results of the test with Ritalin are better than the results without Ritalin, then Ritalin apparently is good for him. If it is good for him, then it follows that he must have ADHD. Apparently, the child is Ritalin-deficient and needs it in his bloodstream.

I suggest that you try an experiment: take a test before and after you have sniffed cocaine. With the right dose of cocaine, you will be able to learn (or engage in other pleasurable activities) for hours, at a high level of concentration. In addition, your self-esteem will improve and you'll feel wonderful! And just in case you think this is a ridiculous comparison, know that both Ritalin and cocaine act by binding to the same receptors on your brain cells, and that labora- tory monkeys, addicted to cocaine, did not distinguish between the two drugs when given a choice for self-medication.[65] Just because Ritalin improves TOVA scores, it does not mean that the drug is the best treatment for your child, or even that it is good for him at all!

Don Quixote backs up our intuitive feeling that TOVA may be the child of a drug company, a clever and wretched way to market drugs.

More on Ritalin

The "medicine" Ritalin and its sisters are street cats dressed in evening gowns. They are drugs, not healers. Ritalin's chemical name is *methylphenidate*, and it is an amphetamine type of drug, known on the street as *speed*. Ritalin, speed, cocaine. Their biochemical actions are similar. The feelings they give their us- ers are similar. Actually, the only 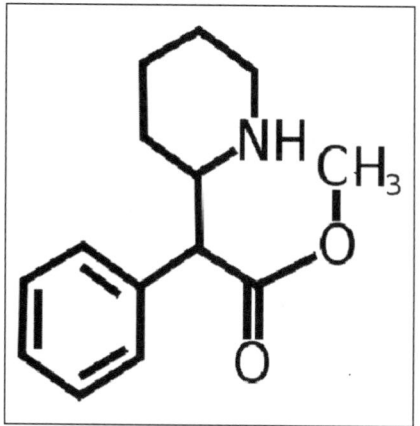 real difference between them is that Ritalin is legal and the others

---

65   DeGrandpre, R. (1999). *Ritalin nation*. New York: W.W. Norton and Company.

are not. Oh, and one more thing: Ritalin is loved and the others are hated. It is loved so much, that parents who refuse to drug their children with it are sometimes accused of negligence. Social workers may even threaten to take their children away from them.

Nerve cells in the brain communicate with each other using neurotransmitters, chemicals carrying "messages" from one nerve cell to another over a narrow space, called a synapse. The neurotransmitter, released into the synapse, binds to a receptor on the next nerve cell and stimulates it to carry the message on to other cells. The neurotransmitter is then released from the receptor, travels back across the synapse and is reabsorbed into the first cell. This process of nerve cell communication is extremely rapid.

Methylphenidate (Ritalin) acts by blocking the reabsorption of particular neurotransmitters, norepinephrine and dopamine, from the synapse, increasing the time they are active and can bind to their receptors again.

Ritalin: Benefits and Side Effects

There is no denying that parents and teachers see many cases of children whose performance in school improves drastically when they begin Ritalin treatment. These reports are important to us because they are numerous.

In general, however, the medical profession prefers to make decisions based on controlled clinical studies, rather than on "anecdotal" evidence — stories of individual experience. There are limits to what we can learn from these stories. First, they are based on short-term observation and say nothing about how the children will be affected over the years. Second, we can't generalize from individual stories to all cases. If I hear 30 times about children who are helped, what about the millions whose stories I do not hear? Were they helped, harmed, or did the drugs do nothing?

Therefore, we want to evaluate conclusions from studies of large samples of children. Here, too, there is a prevailing misunderstanding among the general public, which tends to be overly impressed by any report labeled "research" or "study." So many studies have been carried out on Ritalin, that anyone can find support for his opinion, whatever it may be. It is advisable to relate to any research quoted according to the old Arabic maxim, "Honor him, but suspect him." Of course, this also is applicable to what is written here by your author, a sworn student of Don Quixote, whose exclusion from among the fans of large medical institutions and drug companies is well known.

In any case, we have diligently searched to find a balanced and comprehensive summary of Ritalin research, and behold our selection: *Therapeutics Initiative.* The Initiative is a mainstream newsletter funded by the Health Department of British Columbia (proving that there is no basis for any claim that we are only interested in the opinions of Don Quixote, at least in this case). The newsletter's goal is "to provide physicians and pharmacists with up-to-date, evidence based, practical information on rational drug therapy. The Initiative is an independent organization, which is at arms length from government, pharmaceutical industry and other vested interest groups."[66]

According to the authors, the article before us[67] presents the results of "the best and most relevant studies," detailing both the beneficial and negative results of Ritalin consumption over three time periods: short-term (less than a year), medium term (one to two years), and long-term (more than two years). Before this paper was published, it was sent to 54 doctors and relevant experts for their critique (peer review). The conclusions are as follows:

I. Short-term
Benefits: A meta-analysis[68] of 62 studies examining the effects of Ritalin taken for an average of three weeks found significant improvement in the behavior of the students, as evaluated by parents

---

66   From home page of the *Therapeutic Initiative* web site: *www.ti.ubc.ca/*
67   *What is the evidence for using CNS stimulants to treat ADHD in children? Therapeutics Initiative: Evidence Based Drug Therapy.* Letter 69: March — May 2008. URL: *ti.ubc.ca/en/letter69*
68   A meta-analysis is a study that combines and summarizes the results of a number of research projects in order to strengthen the statistical significance of the results.

and teachers. However, the authors of the meta-analysis,[69] remarked that the results "were likely an overestimate due to non-publication of trials with negative results, and stronger treatment effects in trials with inadequate blinding." (Those who administered the pills, and/ or those who evaluated the behavior knew which child was receiving the drug and which the placebo, thus influencing their perception of the results.)

Harm: The authors reviewed the 10 trials that reported negative events. These were significant, with methylphenidate compared to placebo (a sugar pill), as follows: one out of every four children suffered from decreased appetite; one out of seven had difficulty sleeping; one out of 22 had headaches; one out of 11 children experienced dizziness.

II. Medium term

Benefits: The authors chose a study performed by the U.S. National Institute of Mental Health. Here we see a very interesting statistic, illuminating the extent to which ADHD diagnoses and evaluation is subjective. The teachers involved in the study knew which children in the study were given Ritalin; they were not "blind," and discerned significantly lowered hyperactivity in the group receiving the stimulant. **However, the authors of the study emphasized that when the observers were impartial, that is, "blinded," the ratings between the groups were not significantly different.** In addition, the children rated *themselves* according to an accepted scale[70], and here, too, there was no difference. Most measures of academic achievement also showed no difference.

Harm: During the 14 months of the trial, 49.8% (half!) of the children reported mild negative side effects; 11.4% (one out of 9) had moderate adverse effects and 2.9% (about one of every 35) had serious adverse effects.

---

69   Schachter HM, Pham B, King J, et al. *How efficacious and safe is short-acting methylphenidate for the treatment of attention-deficit disorder in children and adolescents? A meta-analysis.* CMAJ. 2001;165:1475-1488.
70   Mulitidimensional Anxiety Scale for Children

III. Long term

Benefits: The number of controlled clinical trials conducted to examine long-term (more than two years) effects of this drug, which we are giving to so many of our children, is *zero*. The only data we have are from a checkup of the children we met in the previous section, who were reexamined after three years. Five measures of learning which had improved slightly in the Ritalin group in the original 14-month study were checked again after three years. "There were no significant differences between therapy groups for any of these five outcomes," wrote the authors.

Harm: Children who received the drug for three years grew an average of two centimeters (almost one inch) less in height (!) and weighed an average of 2.7 kg (about 6 pounds) less (!) than children who were drug-free during this time

Therapeutic Initiative authors' conclusions

Central nervous system (CNS) stimulants, used among children diagnosed with ADHD:

- improve teacher and parent ratings of hyperactive/impulsive disruptive behavior;
- do not improve children's anxiety ratings, nor measures of their own academic achievement;
- do not improve the incidence of delinquency at three years;
- decrease height and weight at three years;
- have not been studied for their long-term effects on standardized exams, quality of life, school completion, employment, longevity and future health.
- Better evidence of benefit vs. harm is necessary before long-term central nervous system stimulant treatment can be recommended.

According to other sources, only 1.4% of children taking methylphenidate stop treatment because of negative side effects or

because of increased severity of ADHD symptoms. Sleep disturbances can sometimes be reduced by lowering the dose or taking
it earlier. Children who cannot tolerate any dose of a stimulant are
often given an antidepressant drug. These are similar to stimulants,
in that they also play around with neurotransmitters, albeit different ones. Like stimulants, they enable the medical practitioner to
avoid making the effort to search out the underlying causes of the
child's problems. The use of mind-altering drugs teaches a child that
he can medicate his mind. It is not difficult to imagine that he will
be drawn to alcohol and street drugs later on. Ritalin has become
a drug of choice on college campuses, a side-income for students
with a prescription.

Slow-release methylphenidate, the "solution" to some of Ritalin's
problems, is not an encouraging solution, since the dose is greater
than that of regular Ritalin, and the child is exposed to the drug for
a longer time. In simpler language, he spends more hours of his life
"stoned."

Less frequent side effects of methylphenidate mentioned in the
literature[71] include: raised blood pressure, tachycardia (racing heartbeat), vision problems, anxiety, irritability, raised liver enzymes (signifying possible liver damage), anemia, skin eruptions and leucopenia
(lowered white blood cell count, signifying possible damage to the
immune system). At least 800 cases of hallucinations, often involving
visual or tactile sensations of insects, snakes and worms, were voluntarily reported.[72] Claims have been made that taking methylphenidate
has caused enlargement of the heart (and we are not talking about
making the child more generous) and death, as in the story below.

Ritalin: An Internet Report:

As students of Don Quixote, it is incumbent upon us to inform the
public of happenings not carried on the winds created by those wind-

---

71   *Martindale: The Extra Pharmacopeia,* 31st edition, pg.1553.
72   Mosholder, et al. *Hallucinations and other psychotic symptoms associated with the
use of attention-deficit/hyperactivity disorder drugs in children.* Pediatrics Journal, 2009
Feb;123(2):611-6. PMID 19171629.

mills against which we are sworn to do battle. Everyone's opinions and stories can be found on the World Wide Web, and sometimes it is not easy to separate the wheat from the chaff. However, we have no reason to doubt the truth of the story whose URL leaves no doubt as to its content: *www.ritalindeath.com*. We choose to help the parents who sponsor the site to spread their message. These parents were subjected to horrible pressure from people intoxicated by the belief in easy drug solutions to human problems. In the words of the parents:

> We built this website because we didn't want other children to die or suffer side effects because of their parents' lack of knowledge... Since the death of our 14-year-old son Matthew caused from the use of Ritalin prescribed for ADHD, our family has been informing others world wide via the internet about ADHD and the dangers of psychotropic drugs, in memory of our son and countless other children that have died over the years as a direct result of using psychotropic drugs... According to Dr. Ljuba Dragovic, the Chief Pathologist of Oakland County, Michigan, upon autopsy, Matthew's heart showed clear signs of small vessel damage caused from the use of Methylphenidate (Ritalin). **The certificate of death reads: "Death caused from Long Term Use of Methylphenidate, Ritalin."** I was told by one of the medical examiners that a full-grown man's heart weighs about 350 grams and that Matthew's heart's weight was about 402 grams... ***Between 1990 and 2000 there were 186 deaths from methylphenidate reported to the FDA MedWatch program*** [emphasis added], a voluntary reporting scheme, the numbers of which represent no more than 10 to 20% of the actual incidence.

I guess that's enough for now. When considering Ritalin for your child, it is important to know all sides of the story. That is the meaning of "informed consent." It is a health professional's legal obligation to provide parents with *all* the information about Ritalin treatment.

The informed consent offered to Matthew Smith's parents was damaged, biased and incomplete. This is what is given to anyone who does not invest time and effort, choosing to rely on so-called experts recommending the drug. Before anyone gives their child Ritalin, I suggest they take responsibility and study the subject. Statistically, when millions of children are taking a drug, 186 deaths is a small probability. However, for the parents, brothers and sisters of each child among the 186, and for each child, it was 100%.

The Causes of ADHD

Although ADHD is a subjective evaluation, we must relate to these problems seriously. The problems described by the term exist, even though the border between ADHD and not-ADHD is hazy, and they extract a steep price from both the child and society. The price society pays is measured not only by disturbance in the classroom or, in later stages of life, by loss of employment and production, but also by anti-social behavior. It has been shown that more than thirty percent of people with ADHD became involved in theft, more than forty percent began using tobacco or alcohol at an early age, and more than five percent were expelled from school for bad behavior. Similarly, it was found that within the first two years of receiving a driver's license, youths suffering from ADHD caused four times as many car accidents than other youths, and the chance of physical injury in these accidents was higher. They also received three times as many speeding tickets.

Understanding the underlying causes of any disease is crucial to its treatment, so let's define some of the many possible causes of this disorder.

My father was also hyper!

According to *The Merck Manual*, genes are apparently involved in attention deficit disorders. As applied to mental disorders, genetic abnormality usually means that various neurotransmitters, the small molecules carrying communications between cells, are produced in

abnormal balance, and it is this imbalance which causes the disturbance. This concept is far from proven and, at present, we should
regard it as theory only.

It may be that the majority of the general public misunderstands
what is meant when a health problem is blamed on genes. The common understanding, that genes *determine* the physical and mental/
emotional destiny of a child, is incorrect. Genes may influence a
person's physiology, personality and future, but they do not prede-
termine one's destiny.

One of my teachers, Alberto Villoldo, PhD, is a medical anthro-
pologist who spent twenty-five years studying with the spiritual teachers, the shamans, of the Amazon and the Andes. In his book, *Soul
Retrieval* [73], and in verbal teachings, Alberto explains the difference
between fate and destiny. One's *fate* is directed by factors outside
of the individual's control, such as genes, family psychological patterns, family health problems and social environment. Shamans call
the negative influence of fate "the grandfather curse."

Destiny, on the other hand, is a higher purpose, a future based
on free choice. Within each of us is the potential to transcend our
fate and reach our destiny. Our destiny expands before us like rays
of light radiating from a flashlight — many of the rays shine straight
ahead, heavily influenced by fate, but some go off to the sides. We
can change our future by following our destiny to one of the side rays.
Alberto spoke of a friend who was diagnosed with a type and stage of
cancer which is fatal 99% of the time. Alberto told him, "Then you
must change 99% of your life." The man moved to Alaska, fulfilled
an inner desire to become a carpenter and, at last notice, is still alive.

Alberto teaches that if you choose to live according to your fate,
that is what you will get, but if you choose to follow your destiny,
you can achieve anything. This reminds me of a Chinese saying, so
simple and obvious that the wisdom may be missed: "If you continue on the path you are on, you will get to where it goes." Parents

---

73   Alberto Villoldo, *Mending the Past and Healing the Future with Soul Retrieval.* Hay
House, 2005. p. 13. The following is my own loose paraphrasing of Alberto's teaching.

must use inner wisdom to guide their children, while allowing them to pursue their own destiny.

Returning to genetics, we take the broad view. Genes do not act alone; rather, their expression is influenced by the environment, of which nutrition is a major factor. In many cases, the prevalence of ADHD among children of ADHD parents may be due to family dietary habits, parental pressures on the children, the school they go to, and other factors. Even if someday it is proven that ADHD stems from the genetics of neurotransmitters, the genes involved are themselves influenced by nutritional factors. A vast amount of scientific literature shows that gene expression is influenced by the presence or absence of a variety of nutrients. For example, Vitamin D has been found to influence more than 200 genes. The soul influences gene expression, just as it is affected by gene expression, in a two way interaction, a fact well-understood by holistic practitioners. It is a "chicken or egg" kind of thing. Whether a person is sad because his genes produce a "sad" combination of neurotransmitters, or whether the combination of neurotransmitters produce sadness, we must search to find a way out of the cycle, a path from fate to destiny. And there *are* ways.

> *The hen comes from the egg and*
> *The egg comes from the hen,*
> *But I've been wondrin' all this time*
> *Just how it's gonna end.*
> —From an old folk song, sung by Doc Watson

Genetics can also cause heightened sensitivity to environmental pollution, or to factors in food such as gluten in wheat, milk proteins or other allergens. It can be expressed as a greater need for certain nutrients, or in other ways.

In the face of the complexity of ADHD, the medical establishment prefers to ignore many known risk factors and to relate to all types of ADHD as equal, giving them one label, and handing out one prescription. However, when the source of a problem is not recognized and treated, the problem only grows. For example, is it possible for a child to suffer from attention problems because he lacks omega-3 fats, and yet improve when he is treated with Ritalin? Yes, this is possible, but then he may suffer for decades from various states of infection, from low spirit and depression; after age 40, he may develop coronary heart disease or arrhythmia because of the same lack of omega-3. When the source of a medical problem is not found and treated, symptomatic treatment with medicine may allow the problem to express itself in other ways during a patient's life.

The Nutritional Approach

Because it is not specific enough, "ADHD" is not a proper diagnosis. A true diagnosis must point out the cause; once the cause is known, the path to treatment appears. If not, the diagnosis is barren, a mere label. By just diagnosing "ADHD," we might as well call it Idiopathic ADHD (idiopathic = cause not known) and prescribe methylphenidate. I do not consider ADHD a disease; rather, it is a description of children responding to a nutritional deficiency, to our chemically-polluted environment, or to suppression of their destinies.

Many conditions, nutritional and otherwise, can cause or mimic ADHD behavior. Some have been discussed earlier, some are often overlooked, and some are rare. The following is at least a partial list, divided into categories[74]:

Nutritional

1. Hypoglycemia
2. "Malnutrition of the poor" = protein and energy malnutrition
3. Multiple, unidentified nutrient deficiencies
4. B vitamin deficiencies, including B12
5. Essential fatty acid deficiency

---

74   The original list, from which I borrowed heavily, contains 50 conditions mimicking ADHD. The list appears on the Internet, and I was unable to determine the source. Whoever compiled the list did considerable research, and our thanks goes out to him/her. I hope that he/she will be pleased to see the information being spread. I shortened the list by combining some redundant items, and added a few on my own.

6. Iron deficiency or other types of anemia
7. Hyper- or hypothyroidism, often caused by a deficiency of iodine
8. Allergies to specific foods

Certain genetic defects, such as low levels of specific enzymes or slight changes in the forms of enzymes that reduce their ability to speed up chemical reactions, can be compensated for by raising the levels of the coenzyme — a vitamin or mineral, according to the orthomolecular system.

Exposure to toxins and harmful life forms:

9. High lead levels
10. Exposure to a wide variety of environmental toxins
11. High mercury levels from dental fillings, vaccines or other sources
12. Hypothyroidism caused by fluorine/fluoride
13. High manganese levels. Manganese is actually an essential mineral, but can be at excessive levels. (Hair mineral analysis testing can reveal unsafe mineral levels or imbalances between minerals.)
14. Caffeine
15. Worms: these can cause lack of sleep or nightmares that disturb the child's daytime function, or can cause ADHD-type behavior because the child is miserable.
16. Intestinal parasites
17. Viral or bacterial infections
18. Candida albicans yeast infection
19. Drugs, both prescription and illegal, such as the triple DPT vaccine, over-the-counter medications for asthma, hay fever and others

Emotional and learning problems

20. Learning disabilities
21. Sleeping disorders, which can cause tiredness and emotional upset in class

22. Overreaction to the release of stress hormones
23. Bipolar disorder: the symptoms are similar to ADHD. A child can swing from calm one minute to a temper tantrum the next. If a child has bipolar disorder, stimulant medications such as methylphenidate can worsen the condition and may cause psychosis.
24. Lack of exercise
25. Boredom, due to being gifted
26. Gifted and misunderstood: The child is fine, but must learn how to relate to the world around him.
27. High spirit, causing inability to fit society's perceptions of how a child should act
28. Emotional problems of many kinds
29. Lack of communication skills: causes frustration and outbursts

Objective problems

30. Hearing or vision problems
31. Seizure disorders, such as "absence seizures." During an absence seizure, the brain's normal activity shuts down. The child stares blankly, sometimes rotates his eyes upward, occasionally blinks or jerks repetitively. He drops objects, and there may be some mild involuntary movements. The attacks last for only a few seconds, but if they occur dozens of times each day, they can interfere with a child's school performance and be confused with daydreaming by parents and teachers.
32. Various genetic defects that are difficult to uncover or impossible to treat.
33. Tourette's syndrome: typified by facial tics with grimacing and blinking, grunts or other noises. The tics worsen during emotional stress. The disorder can be mistaken for impulsive behavior, not being able to sit still or other ADHD symptoms.
34. Sensory Integration Dysfunction: over-sensitivity to touch,

taste, smell, sound or sight. This could be accompanied by cravings for fast movement such as spinning or rocking, overexcitedness, inattention or overreaction to bright light, particularly fluorescent light. These behaviors may cause the child to be diagnosed with ADHD.

35. Certain spinal problems

36. Head injuries

37. Fetal alcohol syndrome: damage caused to the child's brain by its mother drinking heavily during pregnancy. (High dose B complex vitamins may help in this case.)

38. Inadequate maternal progesterone levels during the first trimester of pregnancy may lead to poor development of regions of the brain necessary for shuttling information and memory and ADHD.[75]

39. Early-stage brain tumors, brain cysts or temporal lobe seizures: all very rare, but, to our great sorrow, must be mentioned.

ADHD behavior may be multifactoral. Here is a description of a hypothetical ADHD child by Dr. Lendon Smith, a famous children's doctor:

The mother was unable to breastfeed him. He is sensitive to cow milk, leading to ear infections with prescriptions for many antibiotics, and subsequent yeast infections. He might have had dehydration, high fevers, inhaled objects, and meningitis. He had all the vaccines, which adversely affects some children. He has eczema, or dry skin. He was put in a walker as an infant, so did not crawl and creep in those early months of life. (Important for later reading skills.) Head injuries are common in the history of these children. He might have had fainting spells or convulsions. He complained

---

75   According to Dr. David Zava and Virginia Hopkins, coauthors with Dr. John Lee of *What Your Doctor May Not Tell You About Breast Cancer.* Dr. Lee did groundbreaking work defining "estrogen dominance syndrome," as explained in his several books.

of muscle cramps or growing pains. He awakened with night terrors. He has Jekyll and Hyde behavior.

Treatment of ADHD

We will not speak at length in this chapter about various nutritional and other treatments of ADHD. Any of the factors discussed in the chapter about FNOBC can cause ADHD, as well as just about any problem dealt with in other parts of this book.

Even though some researchers are not certain, if you ask the field workers — that is, teachers and parents — they have no doubt at all that foods with a high sugar content influence the behavior of children and can cause hyperactivity and difficulty concentrating. When we speak of sugar, white flour products are included. Even though they do not have the same outright sweet taste of sugar, they are just as addictive (witness the drawing power of pasta, pizza, bread and cake), and just as effective in contributing to ADHD. When Don Quixote and his disciples meet, there is always a minute of stunned silence when someone mentions the kindergarten party from which the pure little ones emerged, stuffed with sweets and clutching a take-home bag of more of the same!

Simple carbohydrates must be minimized in the diet of every child, especially those suffering from ADHD. Omega-3 fish oil is basic and should be given to every child with any learning or emotional, any soul disorder. Iron, B12 and blood sugar levels must be checked. Supplemental B complex should be given, and the child should take an adult multivitamin. Magnesium and other supplements should be considered, depending on the individual child's situation, with guidance from an orthomolecular practitioner. Every part of the child's diet and lifestyle should be improved, making changes toward fulfilling the Fourteen Rules outlined in Chapter 2. The list of conditions mimicking or causing ADHD behavior is a checklist, to be used in the detective work necessary for uncovering the problems, and treating of the soul of a child.

Some other treatment modalities helpful in treating ADHD:

- Therapeutic touch techniques: massage, shiatsu, reflexology. Some children are unable to receive these therapies because of extreme sensitivity to touch. In these cases, energy healing, not involving touch, may be used.
- Biofeedback can teach a child to change his own brain wave patterns.
- Bach Flower Remedies use the energetic imprint of flowers on water. These remedies work on deep soul levels and can aid the child with problems of low self-esteem, fears, depression and inability to concentrate. This treatment modality may sound like science fiction, but it often seems effective. The principle is similar to that of homeopathy, which also may help treat ADHD.
- Aromatherapy. The use of specific powerful essential plant oils that can calm the central nervous system.
- Parental support groups. Besides emotional support, important knowledge is exchanged.
- Guided imagery is very effective with children. A skilled practitioner can help a child understand himself more deeply and develop a different relationship to his difficulties.
- Yoga, chi gong, tai chi, martial arts, music therapy, art therapy, behavioral therapy, emotional counseling, social skills training, sports, meditation, connecting to nature, ...
- Love, patience, understanding, acceptance, ...

The final treatment method — love, patience, understanding, acceptance — is universal medicine. The soul of a child is a crystal, and your love shapes it into a beautiful one.

Chapter 9

The Shattered: Schizophrenia

No amount of evidence can persuade someone who is not listening.
                                                    —Dr. Abram Hoffer

Preliminary note: There are valuable general ideas and information in this chapter, so please do not skip reading it because "this will never happen to me." Although not a psychiatrist, I advise people concerning the treatment of schizophrenia. The following discussion is not intended to offer treatment advice, but to play the vital role of raising awareness of the curative potential of orthomolecular schizophrenia treatment. When confronted with a case of this disease, my readers will know that there is an effective course of treatment and will seek it. The sufferer will possibly be saved from a lifetime of torture, which is about all that conventional medicine has to offer. This chapter has additional importance for every parent, as

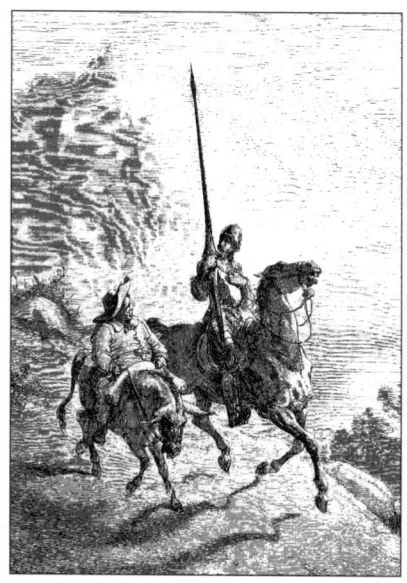

the early symptoms of schizophrenia in children may be similar to other soul problems and share the same treatment. Early notice of these symptoms and suitable treatment may prevent more serious problems later on. Several excellent books on the subject of orthomolecular psychiatry are listed in the Reference section, for those whose interest may be sparked. If one life is improved by what is written in this chapter, your author will be very pleased indeed, having carried the flag to new territories.

The first time I entered the home of a 16 year old boy suffering from schizophrenia, the best description I could think of was "Hell on Earth." The parents in total despair; the boy in his room, yelling, "ants, ants," as they crawled on the walls, huge and persistent, seen only by him. Voices torturing him with messages only he could hear. The cigarette smoke from his room, mingling with the smoke from his unemployed father's chain-smoking, stinking up the house. His diabetic, overweight mother, weighed down by the burdens of her life and the high-fat, highly refined, highly sugared diet she was feeding her family.

The boy had always experienced difficulties in school. Although he was stressed and got into fights, he was getting by, until he got wild one day and the police were called. He was tied up and taken to the police station, pushed around and yelled at. That ignited his first psychotic attack, the result of adrenaline turning sour. When I first saw him, he had gone for months without a lucid day when he could talk rationally. Perhaps every risk factor for schizophrenia was at play in this boy and his family, contributing to his Hell on Earth.

I wish that I could give you what you are hoping for — the student of Don Quixote riding in and saving the day. It didn't happen. The boy's father refused to consider quitting smoking, nor could his mother imagine feeding her family differently. The boy refused vitamins, and his psychiatrist agreed with him — for different reasons, of course. This was years ago. I don't know what became of this family, and I probably don't want to know.

It's not always that bad. Usually there is a rest between psychotic attacks, when the patient learns to function, and his environment may be more supportive and loving. Full recovery, however, a return to being a productive member of family and society, is rare, under the finest psychiatric care. True hope exists for the great majority of patients only when they and their families brush the chaff from their eyes and look beyond conventional drug treatment, to find orthomolecular, nutritional treatment. This chapter will help them do just that.

What is schizophrenia?

Among the various definitions of schizophrenia, there are two outstanding symptom categories:

- dysperception — confusion of the senses, including such phenomena as seeing, hearing or feeling things that do not exist, and
- thought disorder — thoughts do not connect to one another, and/or are not connected to reality (whatever that is).

The disease is "treated" with various mind-altering/numbing drugs that have horrible side effects and do not cure anyone.

It has been said that when a new concept is presented to an audience of a 100 people, 96 of them will reject it immediately — "in one ear and out the other." Only four will be open to the possibility that what they heard is correct.

Decades ago, a wonderful teacher asked me to take off my glasses and describe what I saw through the window. "A house, bushes, a table, a tree…," said I.

"And you, Sam," said the teacher to my friend, "what do you see?"

"I see what Dolev sees," said Sam, "but I also see cups on the table, a bird on the tree and flowers on the table."

"So," said the teacher, giving over a lesson that has guided me over the years, "what's better, a million Dolevs or one Sam?"

So what, if a million doctors have heard, one from another, that vitamins have no value beyond the treatment of specific diseases, and that dosages larger than the RDA are dangerous and wasteful? So what, if 99% of American psychiatrists favor drugs and scorn the thought that nutrition can treat the brain, that vitamins can be used instead of drugs to improve the condition of schizophrenic patients?

I recently had the privilege of walking the streets late at night with Dr. Warren Levin, the renowned physician who founded the first complementary medicine clinic in New York City in 1974.[76] Dr. Levin explained: If a person claims that he is Napoleon, but when you ask him if he really believes he is, he says, "No, but I like the attention," then he is not delusional. He is only delusional if he really believes it.

According to this, claimed Dr. Levin, many psychiatrists who give drugs to "correct" brain function are delusional. They actually believe that these man-made chemicals are fixing something that God made wrong, and are better than the natural substances used by orthomolecular practitioners.

Why is it that psychiatrists have never been able to accept, or even consider accepting, a form of medicine that has yielded incomparably better results than their own treatments have provided? Perhaps these psychiatrists are complex people who cannot understand simple concepts. How can a few cheap vitamins work, when years of psychoanalysis (at hundreds of dollars an hour), drugs (chemical lobotomy) and shock therapy (non-lethal electrocution) have failed?

Imagine that you are in a large city for the first time, looking for your hotel. You turn off the main street to the left, instead of the right, and get lost in the side streets and alleyways, taking dirt paths between houses, going around and around in circles. Will you ever find your way, no matter how much you spin? If you had only turned in the right direction to begin with, you would have gone straight to your destination. Simple.

---

76   The New York State Board for Medicine was so upset with Dr. Levin for breaking ranks, that he was summoned for a hearing. The great Linus Pauling voluntarily flew in from California and testified for five hours in Dr. Levin's behalf, as did Dr. Abram Hoffer from Vancouver.

That's how it is with modern psychiatry. No matter how much a drug company or a psychiatrist researches the side streets and alleyways of the mind under a microscope or on the office couch, if the direction is wrong to begin with, it doesn't matter how complex and detailed they get. (As a patient said to his shrink after two years of psychotherapy, "I know myself better, but I'm still crazy!"). The direction conventional psychiatry is taking is wrong.

Which is better? A million psychiatrists who treat schizophrenia with expensive talk, poison and shock, with a questionable balance between benefit and harm, or a tiny minority of psychiatrists who have proven the worth of their orthomolecular treatments? These men and women are constantly refining their descriptions of the disease and its treatment, so that success rates are improving decade after decade, ever since Abram Hoffer, Ph.D., M.D., began treat-

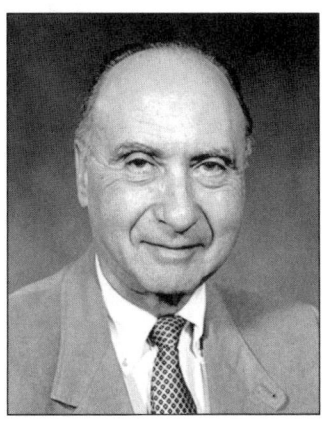

Dr. Abram Hoffer

ing schizophrenic patients with vitamins B3 and C more than 50 years ago. Hoffer has said that there are now seventeen practicing psychiatrists and doctors who were schizophrenic before they were treated by orthomolecular psychiatry!

Miracle drugs

Before talking more about schizophrenia, let's take an historical voyage back to 1747. In that year, Sir James Lind gave sailors in the British Navy a citrus fruit each day. This simple treatment prevented and cured scurvy, a disease that claimed the lives of more sailors than all the other dangers they faced on sea voyages. Men whose bodies were falling apart from internal bleeding, whose gums were softening and dropping teeth, who were dying a painful death, recovered rapidly once they began receiving limes or lemons — miracle drugs!

Sir James may be forgiven for assuming that word would spread quickly, even in those pre-Internet days, that scurvy need never claim another life, and that he himself would immediately become famous. But it didn't quite happen that way. It took more than 40 years and a hundred thousand sailor deaths, until citrus fruit was officially introduced into the Navy's rations, and decades more until it appeared on the menu of England's merchant marine. Sailors on merchant ships died of scurvy, while bringing citrus fruit to their counterparts in the Navy! Hundreds of years later, there still were researchers and doctors who doubted that scurvy was a nutritional deficiency disease, and were trying to find the bug or poison that caused it. Only in the last hundred years, since the isolation and discovery of the exact chemical composition of vitamin C, has the entire medical world finally accepted that scurvy is caused by the lack of one specific nutrient. Even so, the idea that the tiny dose of vitamin C required for scurvy prevention is not the *optimal* dose has not yet penetrated the solid walls of the medical windmills.

It is extremely unlikely that such a simple cause of schizophrenia will be found, a single substance that will cure all cases, the way vitamin C cures scurvy. Schizophrenia is a far more complex and varied disease than is scurvy. However, Dr. Hoffer, the originator of orthomolecular psychiatry, led the way for us to understand that schizophrenia is a disease of biochemical imbalance, caused by nutritional deficiency and/or environmental toxins.

In the southern United States, during the first decades of the twentieth century, and in other places in the world, a disease called pellagra was rampant, killing and disabling many people. The disease was characterized by the "4 Ds": diarrhea, dermatitis, dementia and death. The dementia part filled many mental hospital beds with its victims. Wards were filled with schizophrenics and pellagrins, and it was difficult to distinguish between the two. In the early 1930's, it was discovered that pellagra, like scurvy, was a vitamin deficiency disease. A small dose of niacin or niacinamide, two forms of vitamin B3, quickly cured pellagra. When word spread about this cure, niacin was given to all the hallucinating patients in the mental wards, and many were cured. It was then understood that those who improved after taking the vitamin had been suffering from pellagra. Those who remained sick were still diagnosed as schizophrenic.

The dosage used in those hospitals was not very large, and the niacin was administered for a short time only. At the time, no one thought of trying multi-gram doses and extending the duration of treatment. In the early 1950's, Drs. Hoffer and Osmond developed a theory about the underlying cause of schizophrenia, and began treating schizophrenic patients with vitamin B3 in large doses, usually from 500-1000 mg, two or three times a day. (It may be of interest to former hippies and certain New Age practitioners, that LSD was being used by research psychiatrists to simulate the schizophrenic condition. Dr. Osmond coined the term 'psychedelic'.)

These doctors ran several double-blind, controlled experiments and achieved a 75% cure rate, which was, and still is, totally unheard of using conventional approaches. The timing of these studies, however, was unfortunate. They were published just as tranquilizers came on the scene and were being used for the first time in psychiatric wards. Niacin was a much less attractive treatment — it took more time to work, and there was no money to be made from this cheap, non-patentable substance. The tranquilizers were very effective. That is, they were effective not in curing people, of course, but according to the measurements used in the wards. Believe it or not, folks, the instrument used to measure success was a sound meter! A quiet ward = successful treatment. Don Quixote shouts, "Windmills! They could have done better shooting the patients!!!"

If you want to understand why orthomolecular treatments for schizophrenia and, indeed, for most other medical problems have not been adopted or tried by medicine's windmill organizations, you must look for answers not in the fields of science and medicine, but in those of business and politics. Generations of drug company researchers have developed generations of new tranquilizers and mind-altering drugs in an attempt to ~~make more money~~ treat schizophrenia, yet have gotten nowhere. At the same time, generations of orthomolecular researchers and doctors have improved treatment by defining different biotypes of patients, developing more exacting diagnostic procedures and discovering additional beneficial nutrients and their proper dosage.

Biochemical individuality and drug safety

The orthomolecular approach recognizes the idea of biochemical individuality, best outlined in the classic book on the subject, *Biochemical Individuality*, by Roger Williams, Ph.D.[77] Although the same biochemical processes occur in all humans, and the same nutrients are required to support these processes, there are extreme differences in the efficiency of these processes and in the amounts of nutrients needed for their optimal functioning in different individuals. Williams found that blood levels of various vitamins and minerals differed by as much as 1500% *among healthy individuals!* All-important enzymatic and hormonal activities also vary, as does every human physiological function. Even among laboratory animals, inbred for many generations to limit individual differences for experimental accuracy, there remains a wide range of individual biochemical characteristics.

Biochemical individuality confounds conventional medicine, which seeks standardized drug solutions. It is one of the reasons pharmaceutical drugs are so dangerous. You can never know how an individual will react to these substances, so foreign to human metabolism. Standard measurements of substance toxicity include the "therapeutic index," which compares the amount of a substance that gives a therapeutic effect to the amount that causes toxic effects, and the LD50, short for the Lethal Dose of a substance that will kill 50% of those taking it. The therapeutic index and the LD50 of most prescription drugs do not allow enough leeway for biochemical individuality. Even if no negative effects are noticed immediately, ten years of taking a drug may destroy a patient's quality of life, causing

---

77   Williams, Roger. *Biochemical Individuality.* ©1956 Roger J. Williams; republished, 1998, Keats Publishing Company.

undiagnosed complaints, for which other drugs will be given. Not everyone processes a drug efficiently, breaking it down and excreting it.

On the other hand, orthomolecular substances are, by definition, natural to our human body, which knows how direct them along pathways with feedback mechanisms, breaking them down and getting rid of the excess. The side effects of these substances are actually *positive* in the great majority of cases. Did you ever hear the term "positive side effects" when talking about a prescription drug? Niacin (vitamin B3), the substance found so useful in treating schizophrenia and many other soul disorders, was also the first FDA-approved medicine for lowering cholesterol, after our hero, the same Dr. Abram Hoffer, proved its effectiveness for this! A person who takes niacin to lower his cholesterol might find that, as a side effect, his low-grade chronic depression clears up! And a person who takes it for a soul disorder may find his cholesterol lower. Or, as Dr. William Kaufman discovered in the 1940's, either of these people may find that their arthritis has eased!

Thus it is for all vitamins. Contrary to the view spread by windmills, who are constantly spreading chaff in the eyes of the public about the supposed dangers of vitamins, there are very few dangers in taking most vitamins and some minerals in doses far higher than the RDA, the "Ridiculous Dietary Allowances"[78]. Knowledge is necessary, of course, to avoid rare contraindications, and to get the most benefits from them, but therapeutic ratios of vitamins are generally in orders of magnitude higher than those of drugs, and the LD50 of some vitamins has yet to be reached in laboratory animals. People do not die from taking vitamins. *The danger is in not taking enough.*

Improving treatment

Since Hoffer's initial work with niacin, he and other doctors have greatly improved the treatment of schizophrenia and other soul disorders.

---

78   I borrowed this phrase from the title of the excellent: *Ridiculous Dietary Allowance: An Open Challenge to the RDA for Vitamin C*, by Steve Hickey and Hilary Roberts, 2004. The book is downloadable at *www.lulu.com*.

Vitamin B6 and the mineral zinc are important in treating a specific type of schizophrenic patients. (It is interesting that one indicator of B6 deficiency is the inability to recall dreams. Taking B6 restores dream recall.) B6 has many vital tasks in our bodies and brains. Folic acid and vitamin B12 may be helpful for some types of schizophrenia, but harmful in others. Vitamin C supplementation is important for every human being; in schizophrenics, it prevents the double oxidation of adrenaline, which forms the hallucinogenic substance, adrenochrome, in the body. Chromium is important in balancing sugar. Magnesium supplementation is often vital, and so on and so forth.

One day, when the Lance of Don Quixote finally pierces the walls of the medical windmills, a question may be seriously considered: Is "schizophrenia" a valid diagnosis? If it turns out that the symptoms of schizophrenia are always reactions to nutritional deficiencies or environmental toxins, then a correct diagnosis will define the exact cause. Remember pellagra? When niacin deficiency was removed, so was the diagnosis of schizophrenia. The true diagnosis was "niacin deficiency." If a person over-reacts to a particular substance, causing hallucinations, a correct diagnosis would identify this. An example would be "brain allergy" to cigarette smoke" or to something else. Many patients await the day when their doctors will diagnose them correctly.

Pfeiffer's Law

The knowledge accumulated about orthomolecular psychiatry was used and developed by Dr. Carl Pfeiffer, who achieved a very high success rate in *curing* or greatly improving the condition of his schizophrenic patients. Pfeiffer formulated an important concept in orthomolecular medicine that has become known as "Pfeiffer's Law." It states: "For every drug that benefits a patient, there is a natural substance that can achieve the same effect."

This makes sense. A drug cannot work without participating in a natural process, binding to a cell surface or an enzyme in a place normally reserved for a natural molecule. Instead of giving the drug, we can activate the natural process by raising the concentration of the specific, natural molecule by eating foods rich in it, or by taking a supplement. Psychotropic (mind altering) medicines act by affecting neurotransmitter metabolism. Pfeiffer's Law tells us that we can affect neurotransmitter metabolism using the natural substances from which neurotransmitters are built, or which participate in enzymatic processes. I will explain this further in the next chapter.

Childhood schizophrenia is quite rare. If schizophrenia strikes about one percent of people, and only two percent of these cases begin in childhood, the math works out to about 1 in 5,000 humans being stricken with childhood schizophrenia. Although this means that the risk is low for any particular individual, it does mean that there are approximately 60,000 cases in the U.S. Even more important to consider is that for each of these sixty thousand children, the disease is 100%. It ruins their lives and the lives of those who love them. The hope that orthomolecular psychiatry offers is no less than prevention or cure.

Ignorance or evil?

The closest conventional medicine has come to recognizing nutrition as part of medicine is the acceptance of dietitians into its ranks: *"Welcome to our windmill. Please, please enter within!"* Alongside their drug therapy, many doctors refer some of their patients to dieticians for treatment of problems such as heart disease and diabetes. The dieticians then parrot established lines about not eating fat, and other impotent nutritional concepts, and prescribe a diet. This may help somewhat, delaying the heart patient's bypass surgery or the diabetic's blindness and foot amputation for a year or three. Dieticians will *not* speak of nutrition as the *primary* form of medicine, nor of supplements as a means of *curing* disease. A dietician rarely, if ever, suggests taking a supplement in a dose much beyond the RDA, except in the few cases when doing so is widely accepted. Your run-of-the-mill dietician toes the line and lives inside the windmill. Beyond this, however, conventional medicine has ostracized those who preach the healing power of nutrition — the proponents of orthomolecular medicine, the heroes of Don Quixote and his students — who have seen with their own eyes and presented solid scientific evidence that *nutrition heals.*

This is as good a time as any to ask a major question concerning the refusal of windmill medicine to examine nutritional, orthomolecular medicine seriously: **Is this ignorance, or is this evil?**

Here are just two examples of how windmills relate to orthomolecular medicine — you decide for yourself about the intention involved.

The first is connected to the subject of this chapter: the orthomolecular treatment of schizophrenia. After Hoffer and Osmond found that vitamin B3 is a powerful healing agent for schizophrenia, they conducted nine clinical trials, among which were the first double-blind experiments ever done in the field of psychiatry. The results were overwhelmingly positive about the benefits of the vitamin, and for a decade or so, interest grew among Hoffer's fellow psychiatrists.

Then, in 1973, the American Psychiatric Association (APA) published *The American Psychiatric Association Task Force Report on Megavitamin and Orthomolecular Therapy in Psychiatry.* In this document, the authors summarized the research on the use of niacin for schizophrenia, and concluded that there was no basis for its use. They also claimed that they had asked the proponents of niacin to conduct clinical trials, but that the latter had not done so. This publication, by the respected Authorities of the Human Mind, served to lock mental hospitals' doors with their patients inside, while niacin and its proponents remained out in the snow. In the words of Dr. Hoffer, who was surely one of those "who sees when millions are blind": "The APA bears major responsibility for preventing the introduction of a treatment which would have saved millions of patients from the ravages of chronic schizophrenia. Just as the APA was once captured by psychoanalysis, it is now captured by tranquilizers."[79]

---

79   Hoffer, Abram. *The Vitamin Paradigm Wars.* First appeared in *The Townsend Letter for Doctors and Patients,* June, 1996.

Of the many shortcomings of the 1973 APA paper, three stand out. First, not one of the panel members had ever actually tried to give niacin to a patient. Why was Hoffer, or some other personal witness to the miracle, not invited to participate or advise, if the panel intended to carry out an honest examination?

Second, none of the research papers published by Hoffer was even mentioned, nor was any other positive study. Do you think this was an unintentional oversight?

Third, the refusal of the proponents of niacin to do controlled studies was justified. The studies had actually been done and ignored anyway, so why do more? Even more important, medical ethics demand that doctors give the best treatment they know of to each patient. Totally convinced that niacin is effective for treating schizophrenia, how could Hoffer or others sharing his opinion give a placebo to half the trial participants? Can you imagine a doctor telling you that she knows of a medicine that will work, but, for the sake of humanity, your child may be the one who will take a fake medicine for six months? Withholding treatment for the time of the trial would be immoral for this doctor, against the most basic medical ethics and human decency, especially since orthomolecular psychiatrists had found that the longer a person went untreated, the worse the prognosis. Treating the FNOBC which causes schizophrenia in the early stages enables complete and rapid recovery in the majority of cases, whereas in cases in which the illness has been present for a longer period, recovery may take years, if it happens at all. Those who doubt, but *truly* want to know, *must* conduct trials; those who are already convinced *must not*.

Another obvious proof of the intentional bias against vitamin therapy is seen in the PubMed website, which describes itself thus:

PubMed is a service of the U.S. National Library of Medicine that includes over 18 million citations from MEDLINE and other life science journals for biomedical articles back to the 1950s. PubMed includes links to full text articles and other related resources.

This wonderful site allows any Internet user to enter a virtual medical library and use the search engine to find what has been reported about any medical issue imaginable. Each month, the staff indexes about 5000 medical journals and other sources from around the world, adding many thousands of research abstracts and article reviews to the library.

The International Society of Orthomolecular Medicine (ISOM) began publishing *The Journal of Orthomolecular Medicine* (JOM) in 1970. This excellent and most serious publication has long provided the latest research papers in the field of nutritional therapies. A peer-reviewed medical journal, it has contributors from the top line of researchers and doctors. This journal, however, is *not* indexed in the PubMed library. Pressure has been constant. Every year, letters are written to the selection committee, which refuses to include the JOM in the library, offering flimsy excuses such as lack of funds or lack of qualification according to committee standards. Apparently, the medical standards upheld by the JOM are beneath those upheld by *Playboy* magazine. The PubMed library contains such scholarly titles as:

- Shapely centerfolds. Are women changing or is Playboy?
- "Playboy rabbit" sign: what's your diagnosis?
- Private nurses and playboy bunnies: explaining permissible sex discrimination
- Seven tenths incorrect: heterogeneity and change in the waist-to-hip ratios of Playboy centerfold models and Miss America pageant winners
- Playboy centerfolds and eating disorders—from male pleasure to female pathology?

And Don Quixote's current favorite:

- The prostitute, the playboy, and the poet: rationing schemes for organ transplantation.

Funny, huh?

Some doctors would rather see their patients die than use vitamins.

— Dr. Frederick Klenner, vitamin C pioneer

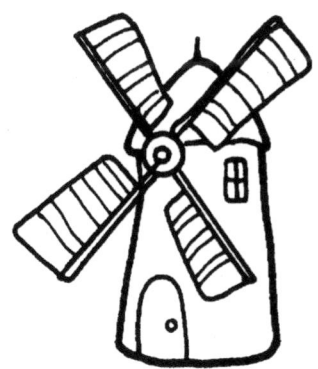

Chapter 10

The Lost: Depression, Etc.

*Too much sanity
may be madness.
And maddest of all,
to see life as it is
and not as it should be!*
— Don Quixote

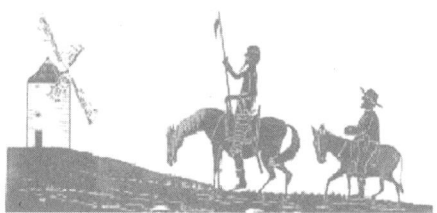

epression is in body/mind. Proper diagnosis obligates deeply understand the forces that lower one's joy and satisfaction with life, the brightness of a soul reflecting the surrounding world. Nutrition may or may not be a major factor in one's depression. A person may slip into soul darkness because she is not living right, not expressing the potential within her. Depression could be a messenger from the soul, blocking the path to mindless living. If the message is understood, it may prevent living out one's life in mediocrity, decade after decade. The depths of the soul do not care what is on the plate or in the bank account; the depths of the soul care about whether ingrained talents are used, whether unique gifts are offered to the world, whether life is being experienced in its fullness and glory.

A child may be depressed because his soul is boxed inside a classroom, while he dreams of hills with story, song and sheep. He may yearn to be a poet, while forced to do long division; he may want to study science, while raised in a family of poets. He may be depressed, because it runs in the family. Being around sad people has taught his subconscious that there is something wrong with being happy; the world is a troubled place, and to be joyous is to be false, to ignore reality. A child could be depressed because of loss or other emotional trauma unresolved, because of belittlement, because of denied emotions.

Standard medical treatment, when the psychologist fails, is to give the patient antidepressant medicines. These act on neurotransmitters, chemicals carrying messages connected to the workings of our soul in a direct, but mysterious way. The most popular antidepressants are selective serotonin reuptake inhibitors (SSRI), which increase the effect of serotonin, based on the theory that the deficiency of this neurotransmitter causes depression. This theory has never been proven. It has never been shown that depressed people have low levels of serotonin and if, in fact, they do, perhaps it is depression that causes a low level of serotonin, not the reverse. Every thought and emotion causes cascades of corresponding biochemical changes on the two-way street between body and mind.[80] When we prescribe chemicals — pharmaceuticals or orthomolecular substances — that affect the workings of the nervous system, we are choosing to influence traffic on this two-way street, hoping to achieve our desired effect of making a person happier.

Real or placebo?

It is not proven that antidepressant medicines work beyond the placebo effect — the belief that the medicine is helping. Belief is such strong medicine that scientists have difficulty believing in the efficacy of any medicinal substance, unless it has been compared to the effect of a fake medicine, an inert placebo. This is why the gold standard

---

80   Two excellent books on this subject are *Quantum Healing: Exploring the Frontiers of Mind/Body Medicine,* by Deepak Chopra, and *Molecules of Emotion,* by Candice Pert.

of evidence-based medicine is a double-blind trial, where one group is given medicine and the other a placebo. The only one who knows who is getting what is an observer who has no direct contact with either group, so that his knowledge does not affect the participants (assuming, of course, that his knowledge has no effect on a meta-physical level, an assumption I make with a grain of salt). This type of trial clarifies the advantage of an active substance over an inert one, by isolating the influence of belief. Placebos have been found to be effective even on biochemical processes that the subject does not understand and cannot feel, and even in cases of placebo *surgery*!

It is an understatement to say "all the more so," when speaking about a mood drug. Belief alone is a powerful healer of depression. In antidepressant drug trials, 35-60% of the patients in the groups receiving a fake drug have improved, just from the placebo effect! By subtracting that percentage from the number of improved patients in the groups receiving the real drug, we find that from zero to 15% of people taking the real drugs have improved because of the chemicals in the drugs themselves. Even this, however, may not be accurate, as the difference may be due to an "enhanced placebo effect." While the inert pill does nothing, the drug may make a subject feel a little funny. He therefore *knows* he is getting the active substance, whereas a subject receiving the placebo cannot be certain. This *knowing* enhances the placebo effect. There are those, such as Dr. Hoffer, who question the validity of using double-blind trials as the gold standard of medical proof, since the clinical situation of a trial does not accurately reflect real world conditions.

It follows that treatment of depression, based on the assumption that a chemical imbalance is the major cause, is on a shaky foundation, compared with such treatments of schizophrenia and other serious psychiatric disorders, where chemical imbalance is more likely. There is no doubt that nutritional deficiencies often play a role in depression, but a complete analysis must be made during the diagnostic process, before deciding to what extent our intervention should center on nutrition or on soul work.

Antidepressant drugs for CHILDREN?!?!

Antidepressants are increasingly being prescribed for children. According to Harvard University's health publication, patients under 18 now account for 5% of antidepressant prescriptions. SSRI-type drugs to treat depression, obsessive-compulsive disorder or anxiety have been prescribed for two to three out of every one hundred children in the United States — more than a half-million children. Figures from the United Kingdom show that four times as many kids under the age of 16 are now taking drugs for mental health problems, as compared to the mid-1990's. Almost 4,000 Australian children under the age of 10 received a prescription for antidepressant drugs in 2007. Of these, 533 were less than five years old, and 48 were babies! Australia has not even approved the use of these drugs for adolescents.

When I was growing up, no one I knew took drugs for the soul. Sometimes, I was sad, and so were my friends. This was accepted, and we were happy most of the time. I remember kicking a stone along the sidewalk for a mile, all the way to school, with a dark cloud in my head. Kicking the stone was partly for the challenge, but my mood was often dark. Poor me, no one offered to drug me. "Being down" was part of life. Night follows day and day follows night. "Being down" is now a disease — an artificial disease, existing even in children, as they learn to deal with what life naturally puts before human beings. Depression has been advertised and made larger than life — to promote and sell drugs. I'm not saying that depression does not exist; it does, and depressed people do need help. The question is *how* to help. Do we throw drugs at the problem, or do we take it seriously, searching for its roots, encouraging, taking proper care of the human organism in which the depression resides, searching out the soul of depression? Life is a deep story.

Really up? Or maybe down?

Following hearings in 2004, the FDA mandated that warnings be printed on the product labels of all antidepressants, cautioning about risk of suicidal thinking and behavior in children and adolescents treated with these drugs. Physical side effects include tremors, twitching, sweating, dry mouth, flu symptoms, nausea, diarrhea, balance and coordination problems, fast heartbeat, blistering skin rash, difficulty breathing, swollen face, lips, tongue and throat, and sometimes convulsions.

On the emotional side — which is supposedly treated by these drugs — the list includes agitation, confusion, trouble sleeping, anxiety, panic attacks, aggression and hostility, hyperactivity (these drugs are sometimes given to children together with Ritalin, even though the combination has not been properly tested, even in adults — so much for the boast about "evidence-based medicine"), and something called "behavioral disinhibition[81]." This curious term is often used to describe what happens to people under the influence of alcohol and other drugs. It is defined as the reduced ability to "edit" or manage immediate and impulsive responses to situations. In other words, loss of self-control. This may be benign, comparable to what happens to people mildly under the influence of alcohol. However, you might join me in my alarm by imagining what could happen when behavioral disinhibition cohabits with some of the other emotional and cognitive effects listed above — especially the aggression and hostility. I'll bet that many of the young people who have gone on murderous rampages in schools are expressing the "behavioral disinhibition" side effects of the drug they are taking for depression. We've all heard the surprise expressed by friends and neighbors after these mass murders: "I never imagined that he was capable of doing such a thing. He was a bit strange, but gentle." Well, he

---

81   Wilnes TE, Biederman J, Kwon A, Chase R, Greenberg L, Mick E, et al. *A systematic chart review of the nature of psychiatric adverse events in children and adolescents treated with selective serotonin reuptake inhibitors.* J Child Adolesc Psychopharmacol 2003;13(2):143-52. PMID: 12886909.

probably *was* incapable of such a thing without being made totally crazy by taking his medicine!!!

Finally, the side effects list includes "more depression." Although the "less depression" drug itself may be causing "more depression," this may be interpreted by the treating doctor as a need for a higher dose, or for neuroleptic (antipsychotic) medication. Nice. Can you say "downward spiral"? Isn't it a bit strange that some of the emotional side effects of mind drugs are exactly what they are designed to prevent? Could we be on the wrong track?

"Mama, don't take my kodachrome[82] away," sang Simon and Garfunkel. My clients have described the effect of antidepressants as a dulling of all emotions, not just the downs, turning their emotional world from colorful to black-and-white. They have complained of loss of libido, of marriages losing their luster. Certainly. If feelings are dulled, the person across the room will look a bit less attractive. For high-schoolers, this may actually be a learning advantage — I can't image how much knowledge passed me by in 12th grade, while I was meditating on the goddess in the front row! However, many adults have reported a side effect of antidepressant drugs not listed on the product label: the concurrent need for Viagra. May our children's paths in life be full of color!

Researchers examined side effect charts from 82 studies of children between the ages of 9 and 15, who were given SSRI medications for depression and obsessive-compulsive disorder.[83] "Psychiatric adverse events" occurred in 22% of the children — more than one in five! The onset of these "events" was seen on the average of three months after beginning the therapy, so they were not initial reactions, which were even more common. Discontinuation of the medication has its own problems and must be done under medical supervision. When an SSRI is started again after it has been discontinued, the incidence of psychiatric adverse events doubles. "The fact

---

82   Kodachrome was the first successfully mass-marketed color film.
83   Ibid.

that researchers have minimized these adverse events underscores concerns about the complex conflicts of interest that may affect the conduct, analysis and reporting of clinical trials."[84]

> The high placebo response of SSRIs may reinforce physician prescribing, and it has been difficult for many physicians to accept that SSRIs may be ineffective... The disappointing reality is that antidepressant medications have minimal to no effectiveness in childhood depression beyond a placebo effect. [emphasis added][85]

Since the placebo effect is so powerful and safe, many times more powerful than the drugs — with their proven risks and questionable benefits— the solution seems obvious. I have a win-win solution: pharmaceutical companies should market placebos disguised as drugs! They could still charge their outrageous prices, doctors could still get rich from their fees, and everyone will be happy. Making the patient pay the high financial cost of depression would *actually have to be maintained*, as this enhances the placebo effect! The new "drug" will be called Plebozac™ or Prozebo™. (I have registered these trademarks, so I'll get a piece of the pie when my ingenious ideas are accepted for the betterment of humankind.)

What about FOOD?

The search for nutritional treatments for depressive disorders took me to the websites of the U.S. Food and Drug Administration (FDA), the Mayo Clinic, the National Institute of Mental Health (NIMH), the Harvard School of Medicine, the American Psychiatric Association, the American Psychological Association, the National Mental Health Association and other representatives of the Great Medical Care

---

84   Garland, E. Jane. *Facing the Evidence: antidepressant treatment in children and adolescents*. Canadian Medical Association Journal • February 17, 2004; 170 (4). PMID: 14970097. Free full-text article.
85   Ibid.

System of Interconnected Windmills (GMCSOIW). Treatments for depression, bipolar disorder, anxiety, obsessive-compulsive disorder and other related syndromes include (in addition to drugs): psychotherapy (talk therapy), and cognitive-behavioral, interpersonal, psychodynamic, group, and electroconvulsive therapies. *NOWHERE* in those websites did I find the slightest consideration of nutritional factors as contributing to these problems or to their treatment. What I *did* find was this glaring statement: "If you're going to put stuff into your body to help your mind, it must be MY stuff, that you buy from ME!!!" Well, that's not really a quote, but it's certainly the attitude. *What about food?* If we consider the possibility that a drug can help, then there must be something biochemical involved. If there *is* something biochemical involved, then nutrition may be helpful. Period. Lack of recognition of this fact is **the** core mistake of conventional medicine.

Any nutritional deficiency can contribute to depression or other emotional difficulties, so every attempt must be made to follow the rules set out in Chapter 2, as well as to eliminate the specific deficiencies leading to FNOBC. Beyond that, to the extent that we accept the involvement of neurotransmitters in depression, we turn to Pfeiffer's Law: *"If we know how a drug works, we can use nutrients to accomplish the same thing."* Using nutrients, we can easily accomplish the same action as SSRI drugs. We cannot take serotonin itself as an oral supplement, since it breaks down in the bloodstream during its first pass through the liver. What we can do, however, is to ingest the molecules from which serotonin is made. The amino acid, tryptophan, becomes 5-HTP (5-hydroxytryptophan), which then becomes serotonin — a rather simple biochemical path. Supplements of both tryptophan and 5-HTP are available today from health food stores and on the Web[86], and have been found to effectively raise

---

[86]   In 1989, after people become ill and several died after tryptophan supplementation, the substance was removed from the shelves and banned. All of the problems were later traced to one contaminated batch from one Japanese company. Despite the fact that the problem was solved and people in other countries safely took tryptophan by prescription for many years afterwards, the ban was not removed. Tryptophan has returned to the shelves only recently, and is now readily available on the Internet.

serotonin levels in the brain. Tryptophan is generally the better idea, since the serotonin level is raised in a more controlled way. The body directs it down different pathways according to biochemical needs, and feedback mechanisms are in place. On the other hand, 5-HTP becomes serotonin more quickly and surely, but the process is less controlled. Using these substances, there is no need whatsoever for antidepressant drugs; these natural substances work just fine and are much safer. In clinical trials, the herb, St. John's Wort, has also been shown to be just as effective as patented medications, and safer as well. Our preference, however, is tryptophan or 5-HTP. They fit the definition of orthomolecular substances — natural to the human body — and they also follow Pfeiffer's Law.

Some antidepressants (NSRI) raise levels of the neurotransmitter norepinephrine, as well as serotonin levels. If an NSRI drug is found helpful, but the patient wishes to be weaned from it to orthomolecular substances, the amino acid tyrosine might be taken in addition to tryptophan. Tyrosine is the precursor to norepinephrine, and therefore works according to Pfeiffer's Law. Tyrosine must not be given for bipolar disorder or any other situation in which there is a phase of overexcitement (mania). Omega-3 supplementation should be tried by bipolar disorder sufferers; it has been suggested that omega-3 functions similarly to lithium, the most common medication given for treatment of this problem.

All of the factors of FNOBC and other disorders of the soul must be considered when treating depression.

It must be stressed that if the patient has already started taking an antidepressant drug, cessation of the drug, even when being replaced by orthomolecular treatment, must be done under medical supervision. He who got your child into it must get him out of it.

Molecular treatment, whether with drugs or nutrients, is at most only part of the treatment of depression. Look to the soul.

Some think the moment is beyond what can change,
they are plain sick and tired, of the hard and the strange,
Taking your medicine and calling it fate,
without trying to change it ~ is the first clear mistake.

Feeling life's problems, its lessons and wrath,
is the first step to finding your way down this path...

—from *www.thegreatillusion.com*, by Victor Kahn[87]

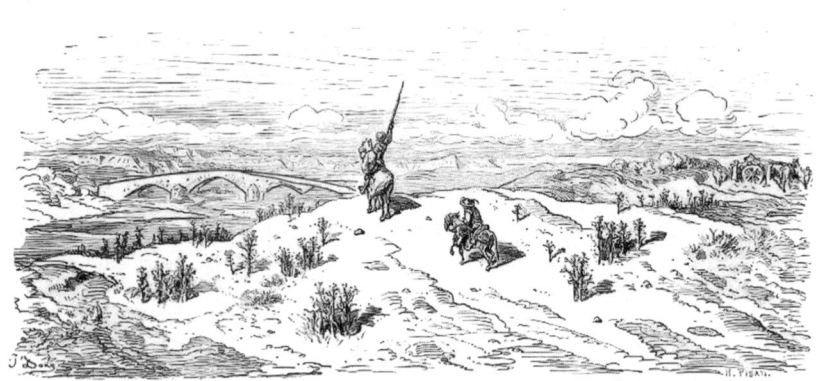

---

87   This is a truly amazing website. Please go there for directions on the path towards enlightenment. These lines from the poem were reproduced here with Victor's permission. Please respect his copyright.

Chapter 11

Down Syndrome

*Medicine cannot **not** study something,
then use supposed ignorance to justify ignoring it.*
— Owen Fonorow

Deep within the unfathomable mysteries of human development, an extra, third copy of a chromosome (a string of genes) sometimes appears — a trisomy. Usually, this change is fatal. One trisomy, however, a third chromosome #21, allows the development of a living human being with certain traits. Although their cognitive abilities are weak, those with trisomy 21 have special talents and gifts, and usually a sweet and open personality. Common physical traits are recognizable: round faces, almond eyes, wide hands with short fingers, small ears and mouth and more. They often have medical conditions such as heart defects, a weak immune system, hearing problems

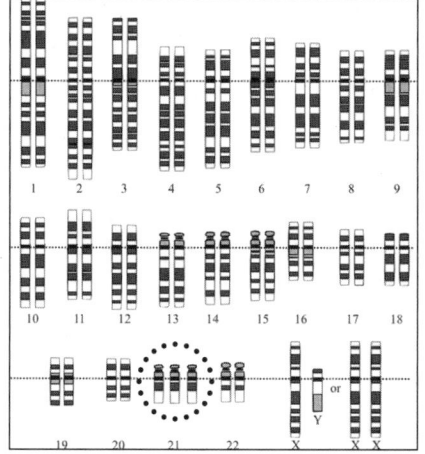

Karyotype for trisomy Down syndrome.
Notice the three copies of chromosome 21
Image credit: U.S. Genome Project

167

and hypothyroidism. All in all, however, children born with trisomy 21, or Down Syndrome, are more like normal children than not. Special understanding and medical care can help Down Syndrome children have a good life.

Can special nutritional protocols help the mind of a child with Down Syndrome? If many have a mental block against treating *other* problems of the soul with nutrition, in this case, the path is blocked by a fortress deep and mighty. Surely, no food can change the underlying genetic cause by eliminating the extra chromosome; however, food, and special nutrients in food, have other powers.

The way genes form a human being and affect growth and function throughout life is not as simple and predictable as transferring ink from pad to paper with a rubber stamp. It is mind-bogglingly complex. Awe-inspiring. Beyond human comprehension. Did you know that nutrients from food, or molecules built from nutrients, penetrate the nuclei of cells and affect the activities of genes? This is the basis for an important term in orthomolecular medicine: genetotrophic[88] refers to the relationship between genes (geneto) and nutrition (trophic). Simply put, nutrition affects genetics.

A "genetotrophic disease" is caused by an individual's genetic need for unusual amounts of one or more specific nutrients. When these are supplied, often in amounts far greater than what can be received from one's diet alone, they compensate for a genetic problem, and ease the disease's symptoms. Having a whole extra chromosome increases the amounts of the enzymes created by genes making up the chromosome. The Down syndrome chromosome, #21, has the smallest number of genes among all chromosomes (which may be why trisomy 21 is not a fatal condition), but, with an estimated 300 genes[89], the complexity is, nonetheless, astronomical. Many of these genes are certainly influenced by nutrients. Therefore, theoretically

---

88   "The Genetotrophic Concept" was originated by Roger Williams, rising naturally from his work on biochemical individuality.
89   Because researchers use different approaches to define the number of genes on each chromosome, the estimated number of genes varies. Chromosome 21 probably contains between 200 - 400 genes. (Wikipedia)

at least, it follows that nutrition *can* affect the ways that trisomy 21, the special genetic abnormality causing Down syndrome, expresses itself. For those among you with scientific or nutritional background, here's a rather technical example:

Chromosome 21 contains the gene which creates the enzyme, superoxide dismutase (SOD), an antioxidant which reduces the superoxide free radical. This free radical is reduced in two steps. First, hydrogen peroxide is formed, which must then be reduced by the enzyme, catalase. Because of the extra gene, a Down syndrome person has extra SOD, so his body chemistry has more hydrogen peroxide to deal with. The gene for catalase, however, is in a different chromosome, so only normal amounts of catalase are produced. The result is that a Down syndrome person is left with extra hydrogen peroxide, a damaging condition! This *genetic* problem can be simply and cheaply treated by administering other antioxidants that reduce hydrogen peroxide, notably vitamin C!

From theory to practice

We've seen that theoretically, nutrition can effect changes in genetic conditions. We will now examine whether, in actuality, nutrition can improve the intelligence of Down Syndrome children.

In 1981, Dr. Ruth Flinn Harrell published a groundbreaking study called *Can nutritional supplements help mentally retarded children? An exploratory study.*[90] The following is her summary of the study results, shortened and edited, with emphases added:

> To explore the hypothesis that mental retardations are in part genetotrophic diseases (diseases in which the genetic pattern of the afflicted individual requires an augmented supply of one or more nutrients...), we carried out a partially double-blind experiment with 16 retarded children (initial IQs, approximately 17-70)

---

90   Harrell and others. *Can nutritional supplements help mentally retarded children? An exploratory study* Proc. Natl. Acad. Sci. USA, Vol 78, No. 1, pp. 574-578. PMID: 6454137. (A link to the free full article is given on the PubMed reference.)

of school age who were given nutritional supplements or placebos during a period of 8 months. The supplement contained 8 minerals in moderate amounts and 11 vitamins, mostly in relatively large amounts. During the first 4- month period (double-blind) **the 5 children who received supplements increased their average IQ by 5.0-9.6** ... whereas the 11 subjects given placebos showed negligible change... **During the second period, the subjects who had been given placebos in the first study received supplements; they showed an average IQ increase of at least 10.2, a highly significant gain... Three of four children with Down syndrome gained between 10 and 25 units in IQ and also showed physical changes toward normal...**

I repeat: *"Three of four children with Down Syndrome gained between 10 and 25 units in IQ, and also showed physical changes toward normal."* To understand the significance of the change in IQ experienced by these children, Dr. Harrell is reported to have commented, "When there was a ten point rise in IQ, the family noticed it. When there was a fifteen point rise in IQ, the teachers noticed it. When there was a twenty point rise in IQ, the neighborhood noticed it."

When asked about whether she had received National Institutes of Health funding for her study, Dr. Harrell replied, "Heavens, no! Nobody knows anything about the area of dietary supplementation, but the National Institutes of Health knows for sure it's impossible."[91]

Before continuing the discussion of Down Syndrome, we must point out that similarly large I.Q. improvements were found in chil-

---

91   Horwitz N. *Vitamins, minerals boost IQ in retarded.* Medical Tribune. Vol 22, No 3. Wednesday, 21 January, 1981. Pages 1 and 19. (From an article by Andrew Saul in The Journal of Orthomolecular Medicine, 2004. Vol 19, No 1, p. 21-26.)

dren with other types of mental retardation. One example was a boy, J.B., age 6, whose I.Q. improved from 54 to 68. He "said only single words such as 'Mama' or 'bye-bye' initially, but could recite, without prompting, the Pledge of Allegiance after 8 months of supplementation and could read the first-grade primer."

The list of supplements given to all of the children is as follows (thyroid hormone was also given when found lacking):

Vitamin A palmitate	15,000 IU
Vitamin D (cholecalciferol)	300 IU
Thiamin (B1)	300 mg
Riboflavin (B2)	200 mg
Niacinamide (B3)	750 mg
Calcium pantothenate (source of B5)	490 mg
Pyridoxine hydrochloride (B6)	350 mg
Cobalamin (B12)	1000 mcg
Folic acid	400 mcg
Vitamin C (ascorbic acid)	1500 mg
Vitamin E (d-alpha tocopheryl succinate	600 IU
Magnesium oxide	300 mg
Calcium carbonate	400 mg
Zinc oxide	30 mg
Manganese gluconate	3 mg
Copper gluconate	1.75 mg
Iron (ferrous fumarate	7.5 mg
Calcium phosphate	37.5 mg
Potassium iodide	150 mcg

Dr. Harrell commented, "It seems certain that better supplements can be found than the particular combination we tested," leaving plenty of room for creative development by future researchers and clinicians. Indeed, valuable work has been done since then in providing supplementation suitable to the newer theoretical and practical understanding of the Down syndrome.

Note that many of the supplements listed above were given in amounts far, far above the RDA doses.

Where truth lies

Since the publication of Dr. Harrell's study, an astounding development has occurred. At least eleven controlled trials have been conducted, attempting to verify her findings. None of these trials have found benefits to Down Syndrome children from nutritional supplementation! The official "Vitamin Therapy Position Statement" of the National Down Syndrome Society (NDSS) says:

> The administration of vitamin therapies (e.g. the vitamin/mineral/amino acid/hormone/enzyme combination) has not been shown to be of benefit in a controlled clinical trial; the rationale advanced for these therapies is unproven; and the previous use of these therapies has not produced any scientifically validated, significant results... Because of the above facts, the National Down Syndrome Society does not endorse the use of vitamin-related therapies.

Not having the treatment protocols of these trials, we do not know if the supplement formulas chosen were similar in dosage to Dr. Harrell's formula, despite the use of the word, "megadoses," in describing the protocols in some of the trials. This word has been misused, and has even described a dose of vitamin C as small as 350 mg., which is considered mega-small by orthomolecular practitioners. Many researchers have reported "no benefits" from vitamins after using doses that even the most lenient orthomolecular practitioner would consider ineffective. These reports would be similar to claims that aspirin, (a standard dose is 325 milligrams) offers "no benefits" to headache sufferers given 30 milligrams.

The most complete review of the clinical trials of nutrition's effect on Down syndrome is a great example of how preconceived notions and bias against vitamins and other nutritional supplements can skew the interpretations of scientific research.[92]. After admitting

---

[92]   Salman M, *Systematic review of the effect of therapeutic dietary supplements and drugs on cognitive function in subjects with Down syndrome.* European Journal of Pediatric Neurology. 2002;6(4):213-9. PMID: 12374588.

that "because of the small number of subjects involved and the over-all unsatisfactory quality of the trials, an effect cannot be excluded at this point...," the author concludes, "Parents of children with Down syndrome should be actively discouraged from giving these 'miracle drugs' to their children." This statement bothers me. The phrase "miracle drugs," as used here, sounds derogatory, an attitude unsuit-ed to a scientific paper, and revealing initial bias. Even worse, if he cannot exclude a positive effect, why does the author conclude that parents should be "actively discouraged"? The supplements are safe and the potential is great. Clearly, this researcher began his review with a bias against supplements. The same bias may have existed in the researchers whose work he reviewed, a bias quite common in those circles. While scientists have a lot to offer, they have blinders on, allowing them to see and believe only the results of controlled clinical trials, and earplugs that deafen them to parental testimony. They are unable to hear J.B. pledge his allegiance to the flag.

We can believe these scientists, and the doctors who believe these scientists, if we so choose, and not believe the thousands of parents who have chosen to walk the nutritional path which has lead them to the joys of seeing their Down Syndrome and other learning-challenged children flourish. Various nutritional protocols have been developed. It has been found that a gluten-free, casein[93] free diet is helpful to many Down Syndrome children. Specific nutrients have been found beneficial in many cases — zinc, magnesium, selenium, vitamins D and E, antioxidants, B vitamins, certain amino acids, es-sential fatty acids, digestive enzymes, thyroid hormones, iodine and more. I.Q.'s have been raised, facial swelling diminished and facial fea-tures somewhat normalized, frequency of infections reduced, growth increased, muscle tone and coordination improved, and speech and social skills improved. More Down Syndrome children have begun to

---

93   Casein, a protein in milk, is difficult to digest. A morphine-like product of improper casein digestion, casomorphine, has been found in the urine of Down syndrome children. (MacLeod, *Down Syndrome and Vitamin Therapy,* (Kemanso Publishing Ltd., 2003) p. 49. I urge parents of Down syndrome children to read this book., the only book I found which does justice to the subject of nutritional supplementation for these children.

manage in regular classrooms. Parents have been "actively encouraged" to use these "miracle drugs" — by other parents.

While there is no accepted medical treatment for Down Syndrome, the nutritional, orthomolecular approach is safe and effective. Official organizations caution doctors about giving false hope to parents of Down Syndrome children. Any parent reading this book, or finding positive information on the Internet, will be infused with some hope. Hope will encourage parents to keep trying, to keep searching for help for their child. Is it better to despair? Is it better to accept the niche prepared for their child in a special institution for the "learning challenged"? Hope gives both the parents and the child an infusion of Vitamin "L," and Love will assist the nutritional elements to help the child. We enthusiastically join the ranks of those who encourage parents to find practitioners who can guide them in choosing natural supplements, which may truly be "miracle drugs" for their children. Do not deposit your hope on your doctor's desk.

It is not the strongest of the species that survives, nor the most intelligent. It is the one that is most adaptable to change that survives. — Charles Darwin

---

Chapter 12

Autism is Treatable!!!
Save the Children!!!

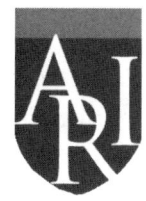

AUTISM RESEARCH INSTITUTE
Autism is Treatable

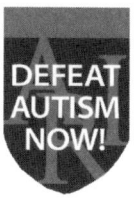

*"If we had just listened to our physician, Our son would still
be autistic, there's no doubt in my mind."*

A utism is treatable." If this is true, why do I need to say it?
Why do I need to write about it? Why is this not known to
everyone, and why are so many children left untreated?!?!

A child frenetically screams and has tantrums throughout most of
the day. At the age of four, he does not relate to his parents, hasn't
had a normal bowel movement in two years and does not speak
beyond a few guttural sounds. Then, he is treated by a varied nutritional program. A few years later, he is doing as well in school, and
in life, for that matter, as any other child.

A second child with the same symptoms is not treated by the nutritional program and has progressed from "gaga" to "mama" during
the same time period. Who is dumb enough to say that the nutritional
program had nothing to do with the first child's recovery? Most pediatricians, that's who! The same pediatricians who told the second
child's mother to keep giving the kid vaccinations, even though he

had severe reactions to past injections, was not developing properly and was obviously sick. Words cannot express the outrage.

If you think a road goes nowhere, you will not walk on it. If you have no hope, you will not try. If you think your child is broken beyond repair, you will not try to heal him.

Autistic children are not defective or broken. They are sick. Autism is a complex disease, expressing itself somewhat differently in each case. It is an expression of disturbances of metabolism, of biochemistry, of cellular function, of digestive tract, nervous system and immune physiology. Although there may be additional causes and genetic influences, the major cause seems to be poisoning by mercury, lead and other metals. The signs of autism are primarily signs of mercury poisoning. Mercury from the vaccine additive thimerosal, from dental amalgam fillings — foolishly placed into human teeth, even into the teeth of pregnant women — spiced with more mercury from fish and other environmental sources. Genetically, some people are 10,000 times more sensitive to mercury than others.

Most autistic children were normal, healthy babies, bringing joy to their families — until the standard vaccination overload struck them, poisoning their genetically susceptible beings. Head banging on walls and concrete, rocking and shaking, spitting and scratching and shrieking — these bizarre behaviors are expressions of being sick, in pain. Autistic children cannot express in words the pain and confusion caused by the poison injected into their vast and wondrous human physiology — mercury atoms binding to molecules in the wrong places, disrupting the symphony. Their souls are tormented.

In 1964, Dr. Bernard Rimland published his book, *Infantile Autism: The Syndrome and Its Implication for a Neural Theory of Behavior*. In 1967, he founded the Autism Research Institute (ARI), a global network of professionals concerned with autism. Rimland's work was instrumental in moving autism from the realm of psychiatry (which maintained that autism was caused by poor parenting — "refrigerator mothers") to the realm of neurology. Since then, the ARI has become a major source of information, services and hope for tens of thousands of parents. I would be extremely honored if, due to reading this book, a parent or two finds hope and a new beginning by dialing the ARI's Call Center at 1-866-366-3361. The ARI also organizes conferences called "Defeat Autism Now!" (DAN!), a biannual think-tank, bringing experts and parents together.

Autism is very complex, and so is its treatment. Almost all autistic children have major digestive problems, causing great discomfort. Because the resulting poor absorption causes many nutritional deficiencies, the digestive tract is the first focus of treatment. Most autistic children cannot digest gluten from grains (celiac disease) or casein, a milk protein. The most

> It's not whether you get knocked down.
> It's whether you get up.
> — Sara Iqbal, mother of Humza, recovered child

powerful medicine found for autism, most often a prerequisite for recovery, is a gluten-free and casein-free diet (GFCF). In our modern world, it is not very difficult to implement such a diet, as most products are marked, and a wide variety of "permitted" foods is available. When your child's fulfillment in life and his escape from autistic hell depends on it, you may even find it easy. The following story will illustrate the power and necessity of this diet. (Most children do not suffer such a severe clean-out reaction as described in this case.)

...the next day I stripped my house of all gluten and casein. I then watched my daughter go through what I can only describe as — like I'd seen on TV — a heroin withdrawal. She lay on the couch for a week, just shaking and oozing some black nasty-looking stuff from every orifice. I would come back from work and my Mom would say, "I just can't watch this one more day," and I said, "You can't not watch it! It's just a diet for heaven's sake!... We're not removing half her brain, we're just putting her on this diet!" And we rode it out for that first week, and then one day I came back from work, and my Mom said, "I don't know quite how to explain this, but it's like a light came on, and that little girl we remember from soooo long ago, I see her in there a little bit!" Two weeks into the diet, I walked outside with her on my hip, and she said, "Our car." And those were the first words I had heard from her since she was 15 months old [at this time, she was 4]. I realized that we were definitely on the right path.[94]

A video of this girl at age 8 shows her, intelligent and bursting with enthusiasm, playing word games with her mother, who had been told that her daughter was in the lowest percentile of autistic children, that she would probably never talk again, and that she would need to be institutionalized before age 10, when she would be strong enough to injure her mother physically.

Are you one of those people who feel a bit drugged or drowsy after you eat bread or milk products? Many experience this. Well, for an autistic child, you can multiply that feeling by a hundred or more. Gluten and casein are proteins which are particularly difficult to digest. If the digestive tract is not healthy — as is the case with the great majority of autistic children — the undigested particles enter the bloodstream and cause a reaction. The partially digested particles act as opiates, drugging the kid as badly as any street drug could. No wonder autistic children have a hard time talking, and thrash around in frustration. The first focus of treatment is the digestive tract — a GFCF diet, along with anti-fungal, anti-bacterial and anti-viral treatments, dietary enzymes, probiotics and other supplements — according to an individualized treatment plan.

Detailed diagnostic questionnaires and batteries of tests have been developed to zero in on an autistic child's specific needs. Chelation therapy, orally and/or intravenously, involves the use of substances which grab and remove poisonous minerals from the body's tissues and organs. Various vitamins, minerals, amino acids, fatty acids and other supplements have been found useful in treating these children, replenishing their depleted body stores and working as pow-

---

94   This is transcribed from a speech given at the 2006 DAN! Conference in Denver. The entire presentation, and many others, can be watched on the ARI website.

erful, safe medicines, healing and soothing the child's body and soul.

It is perhaps incorrect to use the word "cure," when referring to an autistic child who has become as smart and as functional as any healthy child. He is not really cured, as he may need to stay on his special diet, be treated and treat himself specially his whole life in order to prevent regression. The word "recovered" is more accurate, and is used by parents in describing their formerly autistic children, restored to them by the miracle of nutrition, aided by conventional behavioral and other therapies.

Autism is a treatable disease and, although the process is long and complicated, *recovery* is what happens. Today, there are thousands of children who are *recovered* from autism. They go to school and plan how they will make the world a better place. They will, perhaps, grow up to be especially sensitive people, having been forged by suffering. They are true knights of the victory of Good, the beloved ones of Don Quixote.

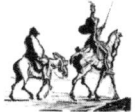

"Some of our families here have been told to put their child in an institution. We're hoping for Harvard!!!"[95]

Hello, my name is Humza Iqbal. My mom wanted me to share some poetry I wrote in 4th grade. Here it goes!:

I Am

I am the grand glory of a first place award winner.
I am a helpful hand that wants to benefit the world.
I am a compassionate heart who wants to help the needy.
I am the madness of a child who is being picked on.
I am the curiosity of a child who is meeting someone new
or learning something new.

95   From the website of TACA: (Talk About Curing Autism): *talkaboutcuringautism.org.*

I am the braveness of a leaping lion ready to attack.
I am the majestic wind, gracefully gliding over the world,
looking at all the new wonders.
I am the sound of love between family and children.
I am a peaceful person who wants to explore the world
and learn new things.

These things help me connect to the world better and to myself.
I hope I can learn new things and more magic can come to me.

By Humza Iqbal, recovered from autism

Hello Dolev,

Thank you very much for your kind remarks. I'm happy to see that you're doing a great service to the autism cause by including info on the biomedical treatments... Thanks for asking about Humza. He's 12 yrs old now, currently in 7th grade (regular school). Thank God he's doing very well academically and socially. He's truly a blessing and a gem of a kid. He has a heart of gold and is everything that is not autism. Back in 2005, San Francisco Chronicle did a story on him, "Chronicles in autism: a boy recovers."

Back in 2005 he had some services, but as of today [December, 2008], thank God he's completely independent and gets no services at school or home(not even an aide at school).

Humza has taught me a lot all through this ordeal and has certainly made me a better mom and a better human being. Whenever I see a kid with autism, I see a "Humza" in him/her. Looking back now, I can't imagine what a gem I would have lost in Humza had I not done anything about his autism.

Regards,
Sara Iqbal

Part Three

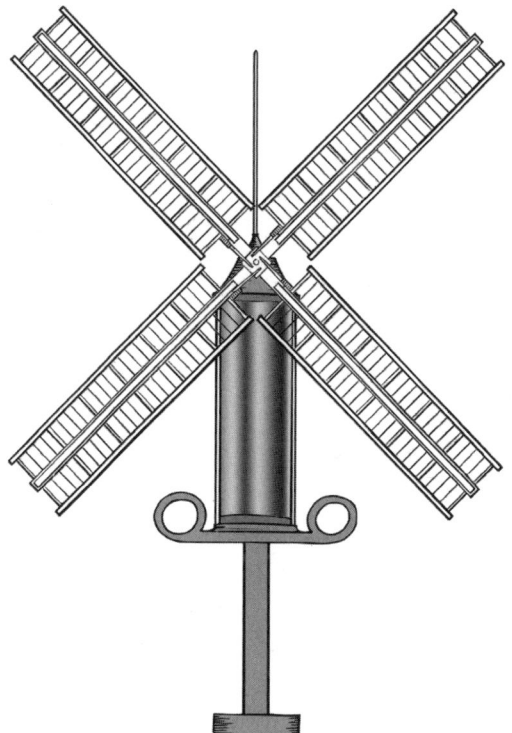

The Good, The Ugly and Some Myth Busting

Chapter 13

The Good: Special Foods and Nutrients

L et your food be your medicine," said Hippocrates, a long time ago. I'm sure you know by now that we consider vitamins and minerals to be natural foods, even if they are concentrated and squeezed into tablets or capsules. The orthomolecular approach defines a molecule as "natural," even when produced in a laboratory, so long as its chemical formula and structure are identical to molecules produced by human biochemistry or used by human biochemistry after being ingested from food.

Natural food will keep us alive and healthy, but we must take special considerations in our modern world, with the nutritional deficiencies and hazardous environmental molecules that face us. In this chapter, we will discuss a few more special foods and nutrients that act as preventative and healing medicines.

Green

The world of vegetation is packaged juice. Cell walls surrounding liquid innards. We can digest some of the packaging material, called "fiber," but not the fiber in grass, cellulose. In the eyes of a free cow, a blanket of food stretches toward the horizon in all directions. We humans, however, are grass-challenged; we lack the enzyme that dissolves cellulose. Nonetheless, we do have intellectual and technical capabilities lacking in grass-eaters. These give us the ability to extract grass juice to drink fresh, or to dry for later consumption.

Wheat grass juice is the best known of these green juices (with barley grass in second place), but there is nothing particularly mystical or unique about wheat grass, just one of thousands of grass species covering our planet. Even more, green juicing need not be limited to grasses. You can juice lettuce, parsley and other greens; many wild plants will release their magic to the knowledgeable. All these plants' juices contain chlorophyll, the green alchemist who turns sunshine into plant food. We, too, benefit from chlorophyll, a true miracle-worker.

Paul Pitchford, in his wonderful book, *Healing with Whole Foods,* lists three categories of chlorophyll's benefits:

- purification: stops bacterial growth in wounds and fungi in the digestive tract; deodorizes, counteracts toxins and deactivates carcinogens
- anti-inflammation: halts tooth decay and gum infection when used as a tooth powder [or chewed]; counteracts sore throat, arthritis and inflammation of the digestive tract, skin and pancreas
- renewal: builds blood; activates enzymes to produce vitamins E, A, and K; promotes healthful intestinal flora; counteracts radiation; renews tissue

Beyond chlorophyll, green juices bring us countless other substances, some known, and others as yet unnamed or undiscovered, which nourish life on our planet.

To get green, you can buy a special juicer with a screw-like presser. Squeeze the goodness out of your green surroundings or out of wheat grass from your local health food store. In that same store, you will also find a variety of dried green products in powder or capsules. The powders cost about half what the capsules do, and give you the idea that they are food, rather than medicine. You can sneak small amounts into your children's food, evading their careful lookout for the new and strange. Many of the products, including "Green Vibrance", which is my favorite, also contain probiotics, vegetable powders, digestive enzymes, vitamins, minerals and more. Some products even contain…

Blue-green algae, such as spirulina and chlorella

The word "superfood" has been used to describe the value of many foods. If I had to choose the winner of the Superfood Competition, it might be blue-green algae, of which the best known are spirulina and chlorella. For the sake of simplicity, I will discuss spirulina, but most of what I say is also true of chlorella and others, although each is unique.

Spirulina is found naturally in warm, alkaline waters in many countries, and has been used for thousands of years. It is now cultivated, and has the potential of alleviating human malnutrition. Name a nutrient, and spirulina most likely has it; name a health problem, and spirulina most likely can help treat it:

> Spirulina… is nature's richest and most complete source of nutrition. Spirulina has a unique blend of nutrients that no single source can offer. The alga contains a wide spectrum of prophylactic and therapeutic nutrients that include B-complex vitamins, minerals, proteins, gamma-linolenic acid and the super anti-oxidants such as beta-carotene, vitamin E, trace elements and a number of unexplored bioactive compounds. Because of its apparent ability to stimulate whole human physiology, Spirulina exhibits therapeutic functions such as antioxidant, anti-bacterial, antiviral, anticancer, anti-inflammatory, anti-allergic and anti-diabetic and plethora of beneficial functions. Spirulina consumption appears to promote the growth of intestinal micro flora as well.[96]

---

96   Kulthreshtha et al. *Spirulina in health care management.* School of Studies in Biochemistry and Biotechnology, Jiwaji University, Gwalior, India. Current Pharmaceutical Biotechnology, Oct. 2008. PubMed: 1588693.

Notably, spirulina contains up to 70% complete protein[97], the most concentrated source known. Beef has around 22%. It is richer in calcium than milk; plus, the calcium in spirulina is absorbed much better and is balanced by magnesium. No toxicity has ever been found, provided that the source is pure. For this reason, it is probably best to buy your algae from a professionally cultivated source, where quality is supervised.

What about the soul of your child? Spirulina can prevent and treat both recognized and unrecognized forms of FNOBC. At least two studies have demonstrated the positive effects of spirulina on children's learning capabilities and behavior.

The first was the doctoral research of Sevulla and Aguirre (1995)[98]. They studied 1,567 school children in a Nicaraguan school, who were given 1 gram (4 capsules) of spirulina a day for six months.

- Teachers reported a 54% percent increase in classroom participation.
- Classroom attendance increased by 21% percent.
- Overall, physical improvements in hair, skin and general health were observed.
- The school's ranking on standardized academic tests went from the lowest to the highest in the nation.
- A dramatic 81% improvement was reported in the children's academic scores.

Claudia Jarratt and her staff at the Harvard Center for Family Wellness (1997) conducted a second study of 142 children, who ate between 0.5 gram and 1 gram of spirulina a day for ten weeks. The results included:

- improved social skills with peers,
- reduced anxiety and depression,

---

97   A protein is called "complete" if it has all the essential amino acids.
98   At the University of Central America in Nicaragua.

- less argumentative, controlling and demanding behavior,
- increased ability to follow directions and focus on tasks, and
- *reports by parents and teachers of significant improvements in children's problem behaviors in 10 out of 11 categories.*

Note that in these studies, only a small dose was given, up to 1 gram, whereas spirulina's maximum effect may be achieved at ten times this dose.

Spirulina, chlorella and other blue-green algae are available in capsules and the more economic powder form. The "blue" in blue-green algae comes from a special pigment that has its own health properties. The "green" is, of course, chlorophyll, so spirulina is a green food, as are...

Sprouts

Baby people are fresh and full of vitality. So are baby plants. Sprouting turns dry, hard, sleeping seeds into fresh vegetables in just a few days. — a miracle that your children will love sharing with you!

Sprouting a seed predigests its nutrients, turning protein into free amino acids and crude fats into free fatty acids, while increasing the vitamin and enzyme content and creating chlorophyll. Sprouts are absolutely the freshest food you can eat, continuing to grow as they go into your mouth! Sprouting is a revelation of nature's alchemy, creating health in your family's bodies and souls.

A variety of sprouts can be bought today in any supermarket and health food store. Alfalfa and mung bean sprouts are the most popular, but if you do-it-yourself, you can sprout:

adzuki bean, almond, amaranth, anise, basil, barley, brown rice, navy bean, pinto bean, lima bean, broccoli, buckwheat, cabbage, cauliflower, celery, chickpeas (garbanzo, humus) chives, cilantro (coriander), clover, cress, dill, fennel, fenugreek, flax seed, kale,

lentils, millet, mustard, oats, onion, peas, psyllium, pumpkin, quinoa, radish, rye, sesame, soybean, spelt, sunflower, watermelon
and wheat.

**Warning! Don't use seeds from packets for planting
unless you are sure that they are untreated. Most seeds
for planting are treated with poisonous chemicals!**

To become a self-sprouter, all you need are wide-mouth jars, a
fine cloth, rubber bands or string, and seeds. Place a few layers of
seeds at the bottom of the jar, add water, fasten the cloth as a cover
and soak the seeds overnight. In the morning, pour off the water,
and then rinse the seeds two or three times a day to keep them
moist (but not soaked). The various seeds sprout within two days to
a week. After they grow a day or two, let them get some sunlight to
increase their chlorophyll content.

Eat the sprouts fresh, add them to salads, or lightly steam the
larger ones to make them easier to digest. If you have too many,
guess what? You can juice them!

You need not stop at "green," so rev up your motors and bathe
your cells with…

Fruit and Vegetable Juices

Fiber is a good thing; a great thing, in fact, just like they say. It improves digestion and moves waste right along from top to bottom. It
is broken down by good bacteria to provide energy to your intestinal
cells. It has cancer-preventing properties. It binds toxins and escorts
them out of our bodies. Low-fiber diets are downright dangerous,
while any healthy diet includes fruits, vegetables and whole foods,
which feed you fiber.

Fiber, nonetheless, can get in the way. Did you ever try to eat
six carrots in ten minutes, with a few apples and a touch of ginger?
Even if you had the patience, your jaw would hurt from breaking up
the fiber. Let your juicer do that part, grinding and removing most
of the fiber (not all) and opening the cell walls to release the con-

centrated mix of vitamins, minerals, phytochemicals, enzymes and more. Juicing fresh fruits and vegetables provides a nutritional bath for your and your children's insides.

Two kinds of juicers can help here: a citrus juicer, which can be hand-operated, and a centrifugal juicer for carrots, apples, squash, cucumbers, beets, celery, grapes, etc. Even a small radish can add some tang. For children, start with some sweet combo based on carrots and apples, and then get them used to other tastes. The fibrous remains can be used in cakes — or fed to your dog, cat, goats or chickens.

Just because carrots and some squash are orange doesn't mean they don't have chlorophyll. Its green color yields to the orange color of carotene, the raw material of vitamin A formation, along with its own health benefits.

Some of chlorophyll's benefits arise from the atom at the center of its structure, the marvelous mineral …

Magnesium (Mg)

Although we discussed magnesium deficiency as a form of FNOBC and suggested its supplementation in treating your child's soul, it deserves extra honorable mention.

Magnesium participates in hundreds of enzymatic reactions, meaning it affects so much biochemistry that we can never understand the true ramifications of its deficiency. Magnesium is deeply involved in the action of ATP, the "energy currency" of our cells. The importance of calcium in humans is stressed by the medical world and known to everyone; magnesium, how-

Chlorophyll Molecule

ever, is mostly ignored, although it is as important as calcium. The two minerals work together, balancing each other. Calcium contracts muscles and can raise blood pressure; magnesium relaxes muscles and can lower blood pressure. Without magnesium, and a couple other factors — vitamin D and vitamin K2 — calcium may settle in soft tissues such as the kidneys and arteries, damaging them, rather than settling in bones. It is generally a big mistake to supplement calcium without magnesium.

Magnesium has been found helpful when supplemented to autistic children, usually along with vitamin B6. Its calming affect is beneficial for children suffering from ADHD, schizophrenia and more. No need to remind me that I said this before; memory is enhanced by hearing things more than once, deepening the neural pathways involved in thought.

Adding magnesium chloride or Epsom salts (magnesium sulfate) to your child's bath water will supplement magnesium through absorption. Foods rich in magnesium include wheat bran, avocado (100 mg. in half an avocado), wheat germ, pumpkin seeds, nuts, oatmeal, soybeans and potatoes with the skin. Chocolate has lots of magnesium, and there are those who claim that magnesium deficiency causes craving for chocolate! That may be true, but personally, I think it's an excuse for maintaining *our* common addiction (notice the humility I demonstrated by including myself). Chocolate also contains harmful caffeine, and is usually mixed with lots of sugar, so, obviously, there are much better things for the brain, such as...

Lecithin

My children and grandchildren call it "brain food." (Hmm, I wonder who gave them that idea.) Lecithin is a fatty substance found in some foods (in Greek, egg yolk is "lekithos"). It is especially abundant in animal brains, and, of course, we *are* animals. Don't worry about that, however. The lecithin I feed my offspring, and almost all the lecithin marketed nowadays, is produced from soybeans, not animal brains. Lecithin is a source of choline, the foundation of the neurotransmitter, acetylcholine, important for memory and learning. Besides the brain food aspect, lecithin helps the body correctly handle fats and cholesterol, emulsifying them for safe passage in the blood and aiding their excretion.

Although the body makes lecithin on its own with the help of some B vitamins and essential fatty acids, regular supplementation is a good idea for child and adult alike. It is available in liquid and capsules, but, best of all, as granules. They are very inexpensive and can be sprinkled into soups, cereals, rice and other grains, stews, etc. For a child with learning difficulties, at least a couple of teaspoons each day is a good therapeutic dose, but any regular consumption should help. Consider it a food, and put it on the table alongside the salt shaker.

By the way, that salt shaker should not have regular salt in it, which is made only of sodium and chloride (with the nerve poison aluminum added to help it flow, and perhaps a positive speck of iodine); rather, it should contain…

Dehydrated Ocean

Man is made of earth and sea. (I'm being poetic here, and could add "and heaven," to include the soul.) One with nature, our solid body holds an internal sea, whose mineral makeup is similar to the great oceans, only at a higher concentration. Unrefined sea salt, in essence grains of dehydrated ocean, can be an important addition to our diets, replacing minerals as they are used. Some consider sea salt a health food, valued as such by *all* the cultures studied by Dr. Weston Price.

Similarly, you can "eat the ocean" another way…

Seaweed

Ocean plants are among the most nutrient-dense foods on the planet, containing all the ocean's minerals, much like sea salt, plus having the benefit of being green food. Seaweed is a healthy addition to your family's diet, compensating for some of the deficiencies in our modern food supply. Seaweeds include nori (sushi wrap), kelp, kombu, wakame and arame.

One of the most important ingredients in seaweed, not readily available in many foods, is...

Iodine

Here's a most misunderstood mineral. For about 200 years, it has been known that iodine prevents goiter, a swelling at the base of the neck caused by an enlarged thyroid gland. Goiter is the most obvious sign of severe iodine deficiency, which also causes cretinism — severe growth and mental retardation. The addition of iodine to table salt, in the form of potassium iodide, was a great medical advance. According to accepted medical opinion, this has provided complete iodine sufficiency wherever the practice has been instituted. This, however, is incorrect.

Goiter and cretinism are only the *late* signs of iodine deficiency, which can also cause thyroid imbalance, precancerous and cancerous changes in breast and ovary tissue (and probably also prostate tissue), learning problems, infertility, and possibly much more. According to the orthomolecular approach, if a major deficiency of a nutrient causes a major mental deficiency, then a minor deficiency of that nutrient probably causes a minor mental deficiency — and we don't want our children to have any mental deficiencies *at all!*

In medical schools and colleges of natural medicine alike, it is taught that almost all the body's iodine is found in the thyroid. This is also incorrect. The thyroid does have the highest concentration, but other organs also have high concentrations of iodine, indicating that they need it.

Potassium iodide in salt is not enough to supply our whole body's iodine needs. The RDA of iodine for adults is 150 microgram (mcg.), rising to 220 during pregnancy. The Safe Upper Limit has been set at 1 mg. (1000 mcg.). The accepted "wisdom" is that more than this amount can block the thyroid's hormone production[99]. Why then,

---

99   Known as the Wolff-Chaikoff effect, Dr. Guy Abraham has clearly shown this "knowledge" to be based on a mistaken interpretation of research data from an animal study, which was then extended to humans. The Wolff-Chaikoff effect does not exist in humans or animals.

is this damage not found in the Japanese, who consume as much as 13 mg. (13,000 mcg.) of iodine per day in the form of seaweed? Japan has far less thyroid problems and breast cancer than does the United States.

Many years ago, when I was first studying nutrition, I noticed a young lady with swelling at the base of her neck. I asked her about hypothyroid symptoms and suggested she get tested. Indeed, she was found to have low hormone levels and was given thyroid hormone as medication. She felt a lot better, but not completely, and never felt quite whole over the years. This is what usually happens when taking thyroid medication, which also causes the thyroid gland to degenerate, since it is no longer needed to produce the hormone.

It was only a year ago that my eyes were opened by Dr. David Brownstein's book, *Iodine: Why You Need It, Why You Can't Live Without It* (2008). Since it has been known for 200 years that iodine deficiency causes goiter, *why are young women like my friend prescribed thyroid hormone rather than iodine???* Iodine is one of the two building blocks of the thyroid hormones, so if there is not enough of it, not enough of the hormones can be built. Hey, that's simple! Hypothyroidism — low levels of thyroid hormones — is a *symptom* caused by iodine deficiency! Why treat a symptom, when we know the cause??? Dr. Brownstein and his mentor, Dr. Guy Abraham[100], have been treating hypothyroidism with iodine for several years, as well as many other health problems, particularly abnormal breast tissue problems, with excellent results. Even breast cancer may disappear.

So, introduce seaweed into your family's diet and, if you suffer from thyroid or breast problems, I suggest studying up on the subject of iodine and finding a health professional familiar with the subject. (The sign is that she won't scare you about iodine excess.)

---

100 *www.optimox.com/pics/Iodine/opt_Research_I.shtml*

The Nobel Prize winner, Dr. Albert Szent Györgi (1893—1986), the physician who discovered vitamin C, wrote:

> "When I was a medical student, iodine in the form of KI [potassium iodide] was the universal medicine. Nobody knew what it did, but it did something and did something good. We students used to sum up the situation in this little rhyme:
> 'If ye don't know where, what, and why
> Prescribe ye then K and I'."

The standard dose of potassium iodide given in his time was one gram, which contains 770 mg. of iodine, about 5,000 times the Ridiculous Dietary Allowance, and 770 times the "Safe Upper Limit." The Iodine Revival is happening. Join us.

Iodine cooperates with other nutrients. Its main companion is found in...

Brazil nuts, the richest food source of the mineral selenium

The thyroid gland produces two major hormones, nicknamed T4 and T3. The numbers refer to the number of iodine atoms attached to "T," the amino acid tyrosine. The gland produces far more T4 than it does T3, although T3 is the active form. In order to remove the fourth iodine atom to activate the hormone, a selenium-containing enzyme is needed. Lack of selenium may cause a deficiency of activated hormone. Selenium participates in the production and use of thyroid hormone in several other ways, as well as having plenty of other vital roles in the human body, such as detoxification (as part of the enzyme, glutathione peroxidase) and possibly tumor suppression.[101]

A Brazil nut has about six times the concentration of selenium as its closest rival, fish. Nutrient tables usually assign about 70 mi-

---

101   Harold D. Foster, PhD, makes a very strong case (which convinced me) that selenium deficiency is the *major* cause of AIDS. His book, *What Really Causes AIDS,* is available as a free download from his website, *www.hdfoster.com.*

crograms of selenium to each nut, so three nuts should be enough to supply the standard therapeutic dose of 200 mcg. This is the accepted view of natural-oriented nutritionists and dieticians, so anyone taking iodine should eat several Brazil nuts every day. In fact, so should everyone else.

That said, if a therapeutic dose of selenium is clearly needed, we cannot rely on nutritional tables, and supplemental selenium-in-a-tablet is necessary. My opinion is based on a research project in which 162 nuts from different regions in Brazil were examined for their selenium content.[102] It was found that the average nut had far less selenium than the amounts in nutrient databases, and that there is a huge "standard deviation" among the nuts, meaning that the selenium content in the nuts is *very* inconsistent — some having almost none. The amount of selenium in a nut depends on the selenium in the soil, which can change almost from tree to tree in the same orchard. In short, Brazil nuts are a great food, and will provide you with selenium, but you can't count on them for a therapeutic dose. If you are taking iodine for a serious health condition, it should be accompanied by a 200 mcg. selenium supplement. Other iodine supporters are B complex, vitamin C and a multi.

Some people worry about the fat content in nuts. I say don't worry about it at all. The fats and oils in nuts are healthy. Nuts are a healthy food. The misunderstanding and lack of scientific basis underlying what the general public has been "fed" about fat, really is "nuts." It's not for nutting that I have placed the following discussion of fats in the chapter called "The Good." Just remember that the truth is not decided by majority vote, as we start our discussion with one of the really good fats...

Coconut oil

Saturated fats are feared. It should be clear by now that we share little of this big, fat fear, although we can't recommend eating large

---

102   Chang, et al. *Selenium content of Brazil nuts from two geographical locations in Brazil.* Chemosphere, Feb.1995. PubMed 7889353.

quantities of modern meat. In any case, if the saturated fats from meat are clearly proven harmful someday, that will have

The truth is not decided by majority vote.

nothing to do with tropical oils, like coconut and palm. A basic understanding of fats and oils is needed to understand why not.

What's the difference between "saturated" and "unsaturated" fats?[103] A saturated fat molecule is a chain of carbon atoms (C), each one connected to two hydrogen atoms (H). The chain is "saturated" with hydrogen. An unsaturated fat is missing one or more pairs of hydrogens on one side of the chain. Notice that this "unsaturated" situation causes a bend in the chain. This bend is one of the two major factors affecting the physical characteristics of a fat and its biological actions.

Straight sticks bundle together much more neatly and solidly than bent sticks. The same is true of straight fats compared to bent ones. Rising temperature makes the molecules move more, causing the bundles to separate. This is the "melting point," different for each type of fat. Eventually, even saturated fat melts to become oil. You've witnessed that when you put butter into a frying pan.

The other important characteristic of a fat is the length of its carbon chain, which may be from 4 to 24 carbons. Long-chain saturated fats melt and become oil at

Saturated

Unsaturated

higher temperatures than do short-chained fats.

In addition to determining the melting point, the degree of saturation and the length of the chain affect the functions of fats and

---

103   For simplicity, I usually use "fat" to include "fat and oil." I also use "fat" instead of using the more accurate term, "fatty acid," when referring to a single fatty acid chain. Two fatty acids join a phosphorus group in the cell membrane. Three join together to form triglycerides. Triglycerides bunch together to form fat tissue.

oils in the human body. This is why coconut oil cannot be convicted just because most of its fats are saturated. Whereas meat has mainly long-chain fats with 16 or 18 carbons, coconut oil has mostly 12 and 14 carbon chains. This makes a world of difference.

Coconut oil, also called coconut butter, has always been a staple food in tropical lands. The populations using it have always been healthy. Lauric acid, the 12-carbon saturated fat making up nearly half of coconut oil, kills viruses, bacteria, one-celled parasites and some types of candida yeast. So does capric acid (10 carbons), which makes up 6-7% of coconut oil. Neither of these damage human cells. Most of what I've said about coconut oil is also true of the other major tropical oil, palm kernel oil.

Fear of saturated fats gave the U.S. oil industry the power to replace imported tropical oils with polyunsaturated oils (having more than one unsaturated pair of carbons). Full-page ads were placed in newspapers by these industries, condemning the use of tropical oils, and on June 3, 1987, an editorial in *The New York Times*, "The Truth About Vegetable Oil," called them "the cheaper, artery-clogging oils from Malaysia and Indonesia." This description is not backed by evidence. Of course, the Malaysians and Indonesians were not in New York to defend themselves. This was a classic case of how commercial interests influence public nutrition beliefs and policy.

The jury is still out, but I believe that, after the test of time, even long-chain saturated fats will be held blameless. Did you know that most of the fats in plaque are not saturated, but unsaturated? How's that for a surprise? And I must say one more thing about fats: *Eating fat does not make you fat!* It makes you satisfied, so you may eat less. Eating too much makes you fat. Eating sugar and such nonsense makes you fat, along with not moving enough.

The more unsaturated a fat is, the more it is vulnerable to oxidation, rancidity. The saturated nature of coconut oil makes it stable. It can sit on the shelf for a couple of years without becoming rancid. This stability makes it an excellent oil for frying your kids' omelets. Margarine, or seed oils — corn and soy — have polyunsaturated fats in them which are destroyed by heat, as well as bad trans-fats[104], and are therefore unhealthy for frying. It's good stuff, this coconut oil, even though it comes from far away.

Olive oil is monounsaturated — one unsaturated pair of carbons — so it is not as stable as saturated but more stable than the other oils. It is okay for frying, but not the best. Olive oil is excellent for other uses, such as salad dressings, and is considered by many to be a health food.

Butter is also better than margarine and seed oils for spreading on your toast or in cooking. Butter fats are about two-thirds saturated and almost a third mono-unsaturated, so it is stable in the frying pan. Butter has a nice amount of the shortest-chained fat, butyric acid (named after butter), which has only four carbons — a short-chain fatty acid. It is highly digestible, liquid at room and body temperatures, and best of all, is an energy source for our intestinal cells. They love it.

Our intestinal cells get butyric acid from another important source. It comes from the digestion of fiber by bacteria known as...

Probiotics

Bacteria in our digestive tract? Yes, four hundred species of them. Zillions of them, outnumbering the cells in your body by ten to one, weighing about three pounds altogether. In each gram of feces there are about 10 billion or so, adding bulk.

These little critters live in harmony together and with you, if you are healthy and have a healthy lifestyle. However, the balance can be interrupted by poor food choices — simple sugars and lack of fiber — and the use of antibiotics. These antibiotics — literally, "against life forms" — are not selective enough, and kill off good gut bacteria. This clears the way for the proliferation of harmful bacteria,

---

104 What is a trans fat? Look at the above diagram of an unsaturated fat chain and notice that two hydrogens, H, are missing on the same side of the carbon chain. When unsaturated fats are heated, some of the chains twist, placing the hydrogens on opposite sides of the chain. This changes the properties and functions of the fats.

as well as the dominance of candida yeast, unharmed by the drugs, the competition for living space having been killed off. The results can be diarrhea or constipation, systemic candida infection, lowered immunity and more. The pathogenic bacteria penetrate the intestinal cells and enter the bloodstream, setting off a chain of reactions and laying waste to the host's wellbeing.

Following antibiotic treatment, it is imperative to use a probiotics supplement for at least a few weeks. **Probiotics are living microorganisms with low or no pathogenicity, which exert beneficial effects on the health of the host.** After ingesting a probiotics supplement, these good bacteria multiply rapidly and replenish the intestinal ecosystem. There, they digest fiber and make short-chain fatty acids which feed intestinal cells, aid the immune system and even create some vitamins.

A wide variety of probiotics supplements is available. Look for one with at least 3 billion organisms per capsule, of at least four types of bacteria — with names like acidophilus and bifidus — since each variety has its own activity.

Sugar is one substance that damages the balance in our intestines. Most sugar substitutes cannot be discussed in a chapter about "The Good," because they're not. One substitute sweetener can be in this chapter, however, and that is the herb…

Stevia

This sweet plant, dried and powdered to produce a sugar substitute, belongs in this chapter, because using it in the place of sugar, the "white thief," is certainly "GOOD." As opposed to synthetic sweeteners, such as the nerve-stimulant aspartame, stevia has been widely used for centuries, and no negative effects have been found. In fact, it may have healthy effects. In fact, it may do the opposite of sugar, by improving the way the body uses glucose.

Stevia is available in liquid and powder, and is much sweeter than sugar. A few drops of liquid or a tiny bit of powder sweetens a cup of drink.

Sleep (Not exactly a nutrient, but I couldn't resist)

"Now, blessings light on him that first invented sleep! It covers a man all over, thoughts and all, like a cloak; it is meat for the hungry, drink for the thirsty, heat for the cold, and cold for the hot. It is the current coin that purchases all the pleasures of the world cheap, and the balance that sets the king and the shepherd, the fool and the wise man, even."

—Miguel de Cervantes, Don Quixote, 1605

ॐॐॐ

When an author writes his acknowledgements at the beginning of a book, he apologizes to anyone he may have left out. There are many "good" nutrients deserving of mention here. I apologize to the ones I left out, and to their human proponents.

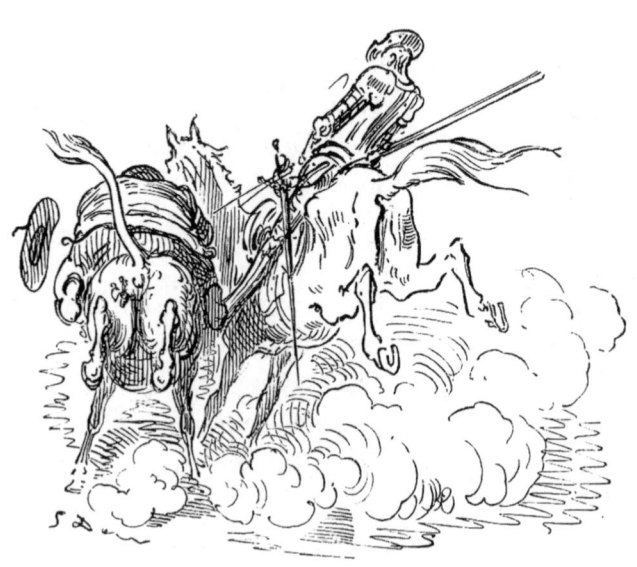

Chapter 14

Living in a Nutritional Minefield

Behold, this only have I found: that God made man upright;
but they have sought out many inventions.

—Ecclesiastes 7:29

Genetically modified organisms (GMOs)

The idea of playing with genes frightens some secret place in my heart and soul. The word "genes" shares the same root as *Genesis*, the name of the first book of the Bible — generation, "In the Beginning." Genes — the codes in DNA, the triple helix at the root of Life itself — us, plants, animals, even bacteria — complex beyond all imagining. What happens when we manipulate the genes which create our food supply, transplanting genes between plant species, or from animals and bacteria into plants? Why don't we tremble? Would I change Shakespeare, and say, "Not to be, or to be"? All the more so, would I not tamper with a code of Life, with a verse from the universe.

Our minds are too limited to play games like these. We are dumb beasts compared to the intelligence of creation. Have we gone mad? Genetically modified organisms (GMOs) and GM foods are uncontrolled experiments that cannot be recalled. They spread their new DNA throughout the neighborhood and change what has always been. They may be fun and fascinating for the scientists involved, with huge profit potential for the scientists' employers, but they are *experiments* with unknown consequences. WE are the lab rats. Our environment is the test tube. It's out of the lab and into the streets and fields, and then fed into the deepest regions of our biological beings.

What is genetic engineering, which creates GMOs? Scientists take the gene or genes they believe responsible for a trait in one organism and insert it into another, hoping the trait will be reproduced. It's a great idea. Create plants with built-in pesticides; implant a gene that protects a plant from an herbicide, leaving a weed-free crop. Create drought-resistant crops. There is no doubt that, *sometimes*, yields have been increased in poor countries using GM seed for corn, cotton, canola and soybeans.

But at what price? We don't know the answer, and the questions loom large:

- Will the massive use of GM seeds destroy biodiversity, the balanced interplay of plants, insects, microbes and animal species?
- Will effective local farming systems, after feeding local populations for hundreds of years, be destroyed?
- Will local varieties of crops be contaminated with pollen from GM crops, a situation that may be irreversible?
- Will insects evolve resistance to a new pesticide-containing crop variety, after its use is widespread — and there's no going back?
- What are the ramifications of letting a company patent life forms?
- What unpredictable effects will appear in ecosystems? Which bugs and plants will flourish and which will disappear? Will a victim be the natural enemy of an unwanted destroyer?
- What are the effects on human health? Allergies? Antibiotic resistance? Unknown results of consuming new plant

genes? What are the health effects of consuming the toxins built into GMO plants?

• Will developing countries become dependent on developed countries, and on industrial giants like Monsanto, the main producer of GM seed? A new type of colonialism?

• Will this lead to the domination of world food production by a few companies? Will they use their enormous financial resources to lobby for the destruction of all competition?[105]

• Will contamination by GM crops destroy organic, sustainable farming?

• What other socioeconomic risks have not been considered? Do the major players in the field even care?

• "Bribery blinds the eyes of the wise and twists the words of the righteous."[106] What research is being hidden by commercial interests? What data has been twisted, intentionally or not?

• So far, GMOs have been used in a limited number of crops. What is bubbling in the imaginations of white-cloaked sorcerers, waiting to be released from their cauldrons once we get used to the idea of Roundup-Ready® corn[107]?

• A recent study[108] has contradicted the long-espoused opinion that Roundup® is safe. Researchers found that various formulations of this Monsanto herbicide damage, and even

---

105   A process like this is happening in the field of medicine. Pushed by the drug companies, the United Nations branch, "Codex Alimentarus," is considering classifying most nutritional substances as drugs. If this happens, they will be available only by prescription, in small doses and at astronomical prices.

106   *Deuteronomy* 16:19

107   A truly ingenious idea was the development of corn and other crops which are resistant to the Monsanto product, Roundup®. This herbicide is absorbed through green leaves and penetrates into the roots, killing just about every plant. By genetic modification, crops are made resistant to Roundup®, and therefore, whole fields can be cleared of competing plant life. Farmers are thus addicted to two Monsanto products: they must buy seed from the company, pay it for licensing the use of seed before every planting, and then buy the herbicide to treat the crop. Quite a profitable arrangement. A life-form has been patented.

108   Benachour and Seralini, *Glyphosate formulations induce apoptosis and necrosis in human umbilical, embryonic, and placental cells.* Chem Res Toxicol. 2009 Jan;22(1):97-105. PubMed 19105591

kill, human umbilical, embryonic and placental cells at even lower concentrations than the concentrations expected to be found in crops sprayed with Roundup®. This is just one example of delayed damage discovery. What else will be found?

- What haven't we thought of yet??? What will the Law of Unintended Consequences reveal?

We don't want to hold back true progress. However, as usual, we are dependent on huge commercial interests and biased governmental oversight for much of our information. Do we want the world's food supply dominated by companies like Monsanto?

Monsanto's website proclaims that it is "helping farmers to meet the needs of a growing planet," "preserving natural resources for future generations" and "increasing incomes and standards of living." A very altruistic company, apparently. Monsanto, with an historic legacy of lawsuits for dumping poisons into water. Monsanto, which brought Agent Orange[109] to the Vietnamese and DDT[110] to the world. Everyone was told these substances were not harmful to humans. Monsanto, a windmill if ever there was one.

The European Union has rejected genetically modified foods for the most part, as have Japan, China and New Zealand. In fact, the standards of many countries are strict, and shipments are rejected

---

109 No need to remind the "sixties" generation what Agent Orange was (is?), but for the younger readers, here we go — A major problem for the U.S. forces during the Vietnam War was finding the National Liberation Army hiding out in the forests. Agent Orange was a defoliant designed to clear forested areas to reveal their hiding places. About 2.5 million acres were sprayed with Agent Orange, something like 5% of Vietnam. It not only damaged trees, but the dioxin in Agent Orange seeped into the water supply and earth, right into the food chain, passing from mouth to womb to fetus and causing chromosomal damage. Monsanto was the main supplier of Agent Orange to the U.S. military.

110 Monsanto was a major producer, but not the only producer, of the pesticide, DDT. In 1962, in her book, *The Silent Spring,* Rachel Carson documented the environmental impacts of the indiscriminate spraying of DDT. This book's publication was one of the signature events in the birth of the environmental movement, resulting in a public outcry that eventually led to most uses of DDT being banned in the US in 1972, although it was exported until 1985.

if they contain traces of GMOs. This has caused economic damage to regular and organic farmers in other countries, whose crops are cross-pollinated from their neighbors' GMO fields. Destruction in the breeze. Cross-pollination has been found as far as 21 kilometers from a GMO crop.

What do the "poor" countries say, those whose populations are supposed to benefit the most from GMOs? Needless to say, the issues are extremely complex, and far beyond the scope of this book. Some of the main issues are touched upon in this description of a meeting in Zimbabwe:

> ...participants discussed fertility requirements, weevil resistance, and environmental impacts. They wanted to know whether the toxin that kills maize stalk borers would not also affect them in the long term, by eating the stalks and the cobs or by eating meat of animals fed on Bt-maize stalks.[111] Farmers wanted to know how Bt crops could affect soil structure, how resistance in pests could build up, and how Bt seed would be priced. There were also concerns about health, religion and power-relations. Participants expressed a general feeling of powerlessness in the face of agribusiness marketing and the lack of government services. According to one participating farmer, *"We may be given seed, or sold it cheaply by companies for a while, but then the subsidy may be withdrawn and we've all lost the varieties we used to use."* Another farmer mentioned the difficulties of controlling GM crops, *"We could talk to our neighbors to try and reduce contamination by keeping the maize varieties separated from each other...*

---

111   "Bt" stands for Bacillus thuringiensis, a naturally occurring soil bacteria that has been isolated and used for decades by organic farmers for control of caterpillars. Bt has a gene that creates a protein poisonous to caterpillars. The genetic engineering folks at Monsanto have transplanted that gene into various plant species. The plants now contain that protein in every cell. What will be the results of ingesting large amounts of it when it is incorporated into every cell of the plant we eat?

but without bylaws we can't make decisions as a community on
excluding varieties."[112]

Devlin Kuyek's paper, *Genetically Modified Crops in Africa:*
Implications for Small Farmers,[113] is an excellent resource for those
wanting to know more about this subject. His conclusion:

> African farmers are skilled and knowledgeable and are responsible
> for the vast majority of agricultural innovation that has succeeded
> in Africa. The low levels of productivity that are often cited in ref-
> erence to African agriculture are the result of poverty, displace-
> ment, war, colonialism, and environmental challenges. Africa's
> small farmers do not need the false promises of genetic engineer-
> ing; they need concrete measures that will attack the root causes
> of poverty and enable them to farm according to their capabilities.

Food supply to the world is a serious issue, and in the case of
GMOs, the judge is just entering the courtroom. There may be light
at the end of the tunnel, but it might be the headlight of an ap-
proaching train. The train may be unstoppable, and GMOs will be
a part of our existence, just as poisonous pesticides are. There are
benefits and there is harm.

Our advice, at this time, is to avoid genetically modified foods
whenever possible. Check labels, especially of soy and corn products,
since perhaps 70% of the corn and soybeans in the United States are
GMO. Although the FDA sees no difference between GMO and non-
GMO food, and therefore does not force the labeling of GMO products, companies with awareness of the issues involved often label their
products "non-GMO." It is a question of offering free choice to concerned consumers who do not want to take part in the experiment.

---

112   Jessamijn Miedema, "Discussing genetic engineering with communal farmers in Zimbabwe," in Michel Pimbert, Tom Wakeford and PV Satheesh, *Citizens' Juries on GMOs
and Farming Futures in India: www.ids.ac.uk/ids/env/GMOsIndia.pdf.*
113   *www.grain.org/briefings_files/africa-gmo-2002-en.pdf*

Monsanto also wears another hat, as the proud owner of NutraSweet, the manufacturer of...

Aspartame

Thousands of products try to seduce you into thinking you can lose weight by using them, because instead of sugar, they contain aspartame or other artificial sweeteners. What a joke to take a bottle of dirty water and call it a "diet" drink! If you buy it, the joke's on you. God, or nature, provide us with *water* to drink.

When researching aspartame in the online U.S. National Library of Medicine, I found that the great majority of studies approve the use of aspartame, testifying to its safety. I began to think that the opposition to aspartame common on the World Wide Web is baseless, alarmist information. I was almost seduced.

Fortunately, I bumped into a review by Dr. Ralph Walton of Northeastern Ohio Universities College of Medicine.[114] Dr. Walton surveyed the medical literature and found 166 studies relevant to the question of aspartame and human safety. His examination of the studies' funding revealed that 74 were funded by aspartame's manufacturer, NutraSweet® (previously named Searle), or related industries, and (surprise!) 100% of those studies attested to aspartame's safety. On the other hand, of the 91 independently funded studies, 84 found that aspartame had one or more adverse reactions. Of the remaining seven studies, one, although independently funded, reviewed only industry-funded studies, and six were funded by the FDA.

One might easily argue that the role of the FDA in approving aspartame has been controversial, and therefore, 100% of independent research has found aspartame to be problematic. There has long been a "revolving door" between top spots in the FDA and the food industries. For 16 years, the FDA refused to approve the use of aspartame in food, based on animal studies showing it to be

114 *www.dorway.com/peerrev.html*

carcinogenic. Then, in 1980, FDA Commissioner Arthur Hull Hayes overruled his own Board and approved aspartame's use in dry foods, extending the permit to beverages in 1983. Three months later, he left the FDA for a high-paying job as consultant to the public relations firm responsible for marketing aspartame.

Dr. Walton concludes that his findings "clearly raise deeply troubling questions, not only regarding the safety of aspartame, but more broadly challenge the current practice of industry sponsorship of research."

Aspartame is a triple molecule. Two components are phenylalanine and aspartic acid, amino acids found in natural proteins and essential for life. Proteins are large, complex molecules that break down slowly; they contain numerous amino acid components which balance each other. Aspartame, on the other hand, breaks down very quickly, releasing phenylalanine and aspartic acid in their free forms. As such, they are nerve stimulants, and have been called "exitotoxins" by Dr. Russel Blaylock, who blames exitotoxins for modern brain diseases like ALS, Parkinson's and Alzheimer's. These substances literally stimulate nerve cells to death, causing brain damage of varying degrees.[115] The third ingredient in aspartame is methanol (wood alcohol), a toxin. Wood alcohol and two nerve stimulants. No wonder aspartame is addictive and good for its manufacturer's business. I watched a very overweight classmate study naturopathy for four years — with a can of a certain cola-flavored diet drink on her desk in every class!

In 1995, under the Freedom of Information Act, the FDA was forced to release its list of 92 aspartame symptoms reported by thousands of victims, including dizziness, tunnel vision and other sight impairment (methanol turns into formaldehyde which damages the retina), disorientation, ear buzzing, loss of balance, severe muscle aches, numbness of the extremities, pancreatitis, episodes of high blood pressure, menstrual flow changes and depression.

---

115 Blaylock, Russel L., M.D. *Exitotoxins: The Taste That Kills.* Health Press, 1996.

You may have seen many people consuming foods that contain aspartame without complaining of ill effects. Don't forget about biochemical individuality — people react very differently to each substance. Some people also just accept health problems as natural, without understanding that they come from somewhere and may be unnecessary.

I hate to say it, but regular sugar is preferable to aspartame. It is less bad. Sugar is also less bad than aspartame's major competition on the artificial sweetener playing field...

Sucralose, brand name: SPLENDA® "Made from sugar, so it tastes like sugar."

Oh, come on, who do you think we are? Just because something is made from something, does it taste the same? Vitamin C is made from the sugar, glucose, but it's sour like a lemon!

The many people who have pinned their rashes, blurred vision, swollen hands and feet, muscle pain, diarrhea, hives and plunging blood pressure to their use of sucralose are lucky, because their sensitivity causes them to stop using it. These are the outward, near-term reactions. The almost non-existent research about deeper, long-term biochemical and cellular influences hints of unfortunate consequences.

Sucralose is not a sugar; it's a chemical that over-stimulates our taste buds for sweetness. The fact is, it's in the same chemical family, chlorinated hydrocarbons, as DDT and Lindane, both pesticides. Perhaps the reason these pesticides are so successful is that they taste sweet to bugs, although I must admit I've never tasted them, nor have I asked a louse for its opinion. A chemical is no longer a sugar when hydrogen/oxygen pairs are exchanged for chlorine atoms. Inventing the name "sucralose" for this pesticide-like concoction (the suffix "ose" denotes a sugar, as in dextrose, sucrose, fructose...) does not change its nature. It just suggests that you can have your sugar and lose weight, too. Naming it Splenda® does not make it splendid.

The manufacturer says that it simply passes through the digestive tract, and that only 15% is absorbed. *Only?* Hey, that's a lot, and independent studies have found greater absorption, as much as 40%! Furthermore, the stuff that is *not* absorbed destroys beneficial probiotic bacteria in our intestines.[116] Maybe that's what causes the diarrhea that often occurs.

They say it doesn't get absorbed into fat. Excuse me, but chlorinated hydrocarbons get into fat, and stay there. The brain has many fat cells.

They say it's 98% pure. Hey, what's the other 2%? "Studies have shown that the final product contains small amounts of heavy metals (like lead), arsenic (rat poison), methanol, triphenolphosphine (toxic to the central nervous system)..."[117]

They say adding chlorine to sugar can't be dangerous. After all, it's an essential nutrient, and we get more chlorine in our table salt (sodium chloride) than from sucralose. They are lying through their teeth. The chlorine in salt is loosely-bound and released as an ion[118], a form used by the body in many ways. Chlorine in sucralose is tightly bound to the carbon chain, a totally different beast. Sucralose and salt are as different as oil and water.

They say it's safe. The FDA does not even require a warning label. But there have been no *independent,* controlled human studies, and *no* human studies lasting more than a year. There is no industry monitoring, just "anecdotal" reports by splendid sufferers. The many, many reports.

Less is known about the last artificial sweetener we will discuss here...

---

116   Abou-Donia et al. *Splenda alters gut microflora and increases intestinal P-glycoprotein and cytochrome P-450 in male rats.* Journal of Toxicoloty and Environmental Health, Vol. 71:21, Jan. 2008.

117   Rachel Naba, *The Bitter Truth About Sweeteners: Splenda's Health Consequences,* The Rising Firefly, Issue 44; (July 8 - September 10, 2003). *theearthcenter.com/ff44splenda. html.*

118   An ion is an electrically-charged particle.

Acesulfame K

"What you don't know won't hurt you," seems to be the FDA's attitude towards acesulfame K (also called acesulfame potassium, sold under the brand names, Sunett, Sweet One and Sweet and Safe.) The FDA approved this chemical sweetener based on the inadequate testing of a German chemical company, Hoechst, the patent owner. No high-quality research has been done on humans.

> I find the actual studies and the data analysis seriously flawed. New tests, properly designed, executed, and analyzed are needed. The usual consequences of poor tests is to make it harder to find any effects. Despite the low quality of the studies reported to you, I find that there is evidence of carcinogenicity. (Marvin Schneiderman, Ph.D. Former Associate Director of Field Studies and Statistics at the National Cancer Institute)

The best attitude towards *any* artificial, non-caloric sweetener is expressed by Michael Corey, Ph.D., in his article, *Splenda or Splendud: The Truth About the Latest and Greatest Artificial Sweetener*:

> **No calorie reduced sweetener is safe. They wouldn't work if they didn't potently and extremely rapidly stimulate, excite, and derange the specialized neurons in the tongue to make them report high levels of sugar when none is there. Anything like this is dangerous to you.**

Do artificial sweeteners = artificial weight loss?

Truth be known, the joke really may be on the consumer trying to control his weight by using artificial sweeteners. These sweeteners may actually cause weight *gain*!

When you think about it, it's very interesting that our weight usually stays steady. According to accepted nutritional wisdom, a pound of weight equals 3500 calories. So, if we cut back only 40 calories a day this year, we will consume 14,600 calories less, and we should lose 4 pounds[119]. Forty calories is the number of calories in two teaspoons of sugar. Theoretically, if we exchange two teaspoons of sugar in our coffee for a non-caloric substitute, that should knock four pounds off our frame in a year. A 12 ounce can of soda averages about 160 calories, so if we exchange *that* for a diet soda every day, 16 pounds should melt off. Sounds pretty simple, doesn't it?

So why is it so difficult to lose weight? Each of us has a "set point," which changes very slowly. Although no one truly understands it, this set point holds our weight more or less steady. We can exercise will power, but not for very long. After reducing calories, our biology overcomes our will, and we eat until we return to our set point. It seems that even if we exchange sugar for artificial sweeteners, our biological set point drives us to eat more calories from another source.

If that were all there is to it, no harm done — no loss, no gain. However, it may be worse than that. In a well-known experiment performed by Purdue University researchers[120] and reported in *Science Daily* (Feb. 11, 2008), rats given yogurt sweetened with zero-calorie saccharin[121] as part of their diet consumed more total calories, gained more weight and put on more body fat than rats fed sugar-sweetened yogurt. The researchers explained, "Animals may use sweet taste to predict the caloric contents of food. Eating sweet non-caloric substances may degrade this predictive relationship..." In other words, our attempt to fool our sense of taste may backfire by confusing our set point mechanism.

Whether or not we can extrapolate from this experiment and say that artificial sweeteners cause us humans to *gain* weight, there is no evidence that they help us *lose* weight. Foods made with no-calorie sweeteners may not be as satisfying as foods made with sugar, and so we eat more of other things. The general population

---

119   The numbers used in these calculations are rounded off for clarity.

120   Davidson and Swithers, *A role for sweet taste: calorie predictive relations in energy regulation by rats.* Behavioral Neuroscience, 2008 Feb; 122 (1):161-73. PubMed 18298259

121   I did not include a discussion of saccharin because its negative effects are generally known, and it has been mostly replaced by other sweeteners.

has certainly not lost weight since the spread of artificial sweeteners — just the opposite. Do you know anyone who has lost weight simply by using them?

In short, "diet drinks" are not diet drinks. *Water*, now *there's* a diet drink. Zero calories and essential for every cell. Cheap, too. For weight loss, use the "Water and Walk" system.

Another commonly used taste additive that joins artificial sweeteners in the club of harmful, allergenic, weight-gain-causing substances is ...

Monosodium glutamate (MSG)

You've probably heard of Chinese Restaurant Syndrome, a list of symptoms — burning sensations in the upper body, facial flushing and numbness, chest pain and heart palpitations, nausea, headache, sweating and wheezing — caused by eating monosodium glutamate. It's not fair to blame this syndrome on Chinese restaurants. At least there you can request that MSG not be added to the food. Not so in American restaurants, where the staff may not even know that there is MSG in the raw materials bought from their suppliers. In fact, it may be more accurate to call it American Diet Syndrome, since MSG is so common in prepared foods.

MSG, like aspartame, contains a natural amino acid, which in its unbalanced, free form is an exitotoxin. MSG is the largest source of exitotoxins in our food supply. Glutamate receptors are found in many parts of the body, including the brain. Brain stimulation, coupled with taste stimulation, make MSG addictive, at least psychologically (it's delicious). People who consume a lot of foods containing MSG find that foods without it are not very flavorful. That's good for the food industry and bad for people.

Other suspected dangers of MSG are heart arrhythmia (which can lead to heart attacks), childhood asthma, insomnia, and damage to blood vessels, ovaries and the pancreas (contributing to diabetes). Many cancers have receptors for glutamate, which may act like tumor fertilizer.

MSG triggers obesity. Babies and small children are more sensitive to it than adults. Baby formulas usually contain soy protein, which breaks down to glutamate and related exitotoxins.

Monosodium glutamate is one of the most common food additives in the U.S. At its side, in the nutritional minefield of the modern supermarket, we are faced with …

Artificial everything

Let's talk about colors, those light waves that hit our retinas and make the world a beautiful place. You have but to open your eyes and wonder at the colors of a carrot, a tomato, an orange, a blade of grass. The wonders of colorful vegetable skins that package food inside, preserving it without refrigeration. These colors are real. Their molecules are health-giving. They are part of our food chain. But what happens to the human body and soul, when natural yellow is faked by using the synthetic molecule, tartrazine (E102, Yellow #5), or green is faked by mixing yellow tartrazine with Brilliant Blue (E133) or Green S (E142) to create shades of green? What happens when unnatural, non-food chemical colors are poured onto a bottle of fizzy, sweet water? What happens when preservatives replace the miracle of fruit skins?

The sad and appalling answer is, we don't know nearly enough. The more we know, the less appealing the use of artificial everything is getting. We *do* know, for example, that tartrazine causes allergic reactions in many people. Sometimes the cause is undetected, since reactions can take a few days to develop.

Dr. Ben Feingold wrote a book called *Why Your Child is Hyperactive* (Random House, 1974), one of the first sources of information about the effects of synthetic food colorings, flavors and other chemical additives on the child's soul. Feingold found that ADHD children improved when put on strict diets, eating only natural foods, free of chemical additives.

Preservatives keep food from breaking down. Well, friends, food is *supposed* to break down, once it passes our teeth. It's called "digestion." Do preservatives interfere with the work of our digestive enzymes, beginning with those in our saliva and continuing in our stomachs and intestines? What do preservatives do in our blood-stream and in our cells? Here we go again, playing games, throwing monkey wrenches into our machinery.

This chapter could go on, and on, and on, but I'm sure you get the idea.

About thirty years ago, I saw a small item in *The Farmers' Almanac*. Undertakers claimed, the article said, that bodies were lasting much longer than they used to, because of the preservatives consumed in modern food.

I think they meant that as a joke, but I'm not sure...

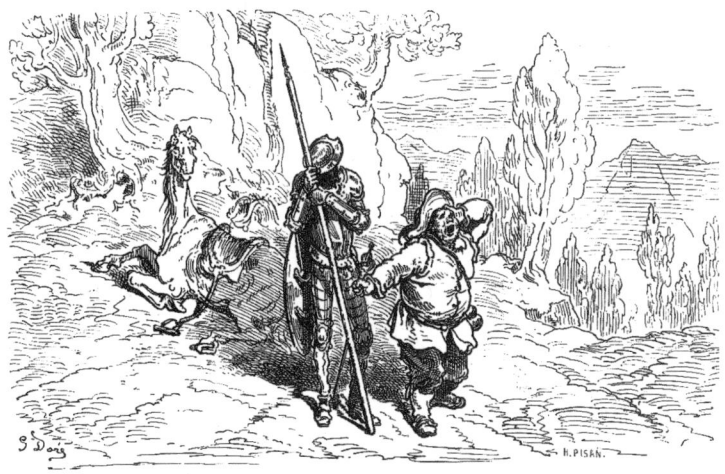

1,501,430,636,558,496,585,414 and the Soul of Your Child

S orry, I'll put it into words: one sextillion, five hundred and one quadrillion, four hundred and thirty trillion, five hundred and fifty eight billion, four hundred and ninety six million, five hundred and eighty five thousand, four hundred and fourteen. *Exactly.*

Nice number? Not. It is the exact number of mercury atoms in half a gram, which is approximately, but not exactly (what's a few quadrillion atoms between friends?) the weight of the mercury in one amalgam filling in your tooth. Each of those atoms, if it escapes from the filling and is absorbed or swallowed or breathed into the bloodstream, has the potential of disrupting the work of an enzyme or another vital molecule in your body. Mercury is perhaps the most poisonous atom in the world.

Your dentist will tell you that the metals in the filling are stable, that you have no mercury exposure. She gets her education from the wrong people — from marketers and others who, for various reasons, want her to think that her methods are safe. And she wants to believe it. All it would take is ten minutes of her time, in

---

122 Some of the information here and several of the research studies quoted were found in the article: *Assessment of Mercury Exposure and Risks from Dental Amalgam.* G. Mark Richardson, Ph.D., Medical Devices Bureau, Environmental Health Directorate, Health Canada August 18, 1995.

the safety of her office, to enter the virtual National Public Library of Medicine (search: "pubmed") on the Internet, to learn that she is mistaken. Her methods are not safe. In fact, amalgam fillings are poisoning her clients, especially the children — and even unborn ones, if she is placing amalgam fillings in pregnant women. The degree of mercury poisoning from amalgam is debatable, and *is* being debated. Some believe that it is *extremely* harmful, while others minimize their estimates of damage. I found, however, *no* sources who used research to base the opinion that mercury is not released from fillings. Your dentist could know that there is a major question here after ten minutes, and could become quite knowledgeable on this subject in a couple of hours.

One might be excused for expecting their dentist to do this; after all, she receives strict safety instructions with the amalgam. She handles it with gloves and great care, so as not to be exposed to it. She must dispose of remains in specific ways, so that the mercury does not become an environmental hazard. She then puts this stuff into *your* mouth. You would think that the American Dental Association (ADA), that windmill of toothy knowledge, would provide mandatory educational seminars about the mercury in amalgam.

Innocent until proven guilty?

To be fair, I must tell you that the ADA has not *completely* ignored the subject. It has only ignored *negative* findings. Its position paper from July, 2008 states:

> Dental amalgam (silver filling) is considered a safe, affordable and durable material that has been used to restore the teeth of more than 100 million Americans. It contains a mixture of metals such as silver, copper and tin, in addition to mercury, which binds these components into a hard, stable and safe substance. Dental amalgam has been studied and reviewed extensively, and has established a record of safety and effectiveness."

We question these conclusions. The maxim, "innocent until proven guilty" can be applied when the suspect is clear of guilt to begin with. Mercury is not. Mercury is a known poison. A vitamin can be considered innocent until proven guilty, and placed in the mouth until clear doubt is raised about its innocence. Mercury is a known vicious poison and is guilty until proven innocent. It is *known* that vapor is released and inhaled. It is *known* that mercury is dissolved from amalgams into saliva. It should not be placed in a human mouth until proven innocent. The ADA paper says, "No controlled studies have been published demonstrating systemic adverse effects from amalgam restorations." In other words, innocent until proven guilty. What kind of studies are they talking about that would satisfy them? Controlled? Should we conduct a study which puts 10 real amalgam fillings into five hundred mouths, and 10 fake, placebo fillings that look like amalgam into five hundred other mouths, and then compare the health of all the participants for 30 years? Would you participate in such a study? If so, send your name to the ADA.

Can you imagine the American Dental Association ever coming out with a statement like: "We hereby inform the public that due to recent discovery, we will no longer be putting amalgam into your mouths because we have now realized that we have poisoned countless millions of people for the last two hundred years"? Dentists will be the last to allow the knowledge of the poisonous power of "silver" fillings to penetrate their windmill walls, so look elsewhere for your information. And they call *us* quacks!

In truth, several countries have already woken up and outlawed the use of amalgam in fillings. These include Germany and Sweden (the Swedish government has apologized for any harm previous fillings may have caused). Other countries have restricted its use, allowing it to poison non-pregnant adults only. The once largest amalgam producer, the Degussa company of Germany, closed down its amalgam division entirely, even though it provided half the company's profits. Good morning, America and Canada and other amalgam-loving and child-ignoring governments! Don Quixote knows who you are and where you live!

> "It is easy to see," replied Don Quixote, "that thou art not used to this business of adventures; those are giants; and if thou art afraid, away with thee out of this and betake thyself to prayer while I engage them in fierce and unequal combat."
>
> So saying, he gave the spur to his steed Rocinante, heedless of the cries his squire Sancho sent after him, warning him...He made at them shouting, "Fly not, cowards and vile beings, for a single knight attacks you."

A "silver" filling is 50% mercury, 35% silver, 9% tin and 6% copper. The vast majority of recent studies have found that mercury is released the entire time the amalgam filling is in the mouth, resulting in constant exposure. This mercury is in a fat-soluble form, so it passes through cell membranes and through the filter known as the blood-brain barrier. Once inside the brain, part of it is converted to a form that does not easily pass through this barrier, so it stays trapped inside the brain for thirty years or so[123],[124].

"A record of safety"
The only questions are about the degree of exposure and whether it causes harm. It has been long assumed — mercury amalgams have been used for 200 years — that since negative effects have not been seen, there is no danger. However, it is only recently that sensitive methods of detecting neurological and other damages have been developed. Acute exposure to poisons is easy to see — the person dies or gets sick immediately after exposure — but chronic, low-level

---

123 Lorscheider, F.L., Vimy, M.J., Penergrass, J.C., Haley, B.E. 1995b. *Mercury vapor exposure inhibits tubulin binding to GTP in rat brain: a molecular lesion also present in human Alzheimer brain.* Presented at: FASEB Annual Meeting, Atlanta, GA, April 12, 1995.
124 Bernard, S.R., Purdue, P. 1984. *Metabolic models for methyl and inorganic mercury.* Halth Phys., 46(3):695-699.

exposure can cause such a wide variety of symptoms that it is difficult to diagnose. Millions of people may have suffered diminished health because of amalgam fillings, but the cause has been hidden. According to the Environmental Protection Agency, the variety of symptoms caused by mercury includes: impairment of peripheral vision; disturbances in sensations like numbness ("pins and needles"), usually in the hands and feet and sometimes around the mouth; lack of coordination; impairment of speech, hearing and walking; skin rashes; mood swings; memory loss and mental disturbance. Other sources continue (we'll make the print smaller and squeeze lines to save space, since we doubt if you will get through the whole list anyway. We do, however, recommend reading it slowly and out loud for maximum effect):

From the British Medical Journal (Waldron, 1961): timidity, diffidence, increasing shyness, loss of self-confidence, anxiety, and a desire to remain unobserved and unobtrusive." Various other sources add: irritability, fearfulness, fits of anger, inability to concentrate, lethargy, insomnia, depression, suicidal tendencies, manic depression, hallucinations and rapid progression of all schizophrenic symptoms, muscle weakness, muscle nerve transmission failure resembling myasthenia gravis, motor neuron disease (ALS), Alzheimer's disease, multiple sclerosis, learning disabilities, autism, neurotransmitter imbalance (interference with metabolism at nerve ends), damage to the blood-brain barrier (allowing the wrong chemicals to visit the brain), bleeding gums, alveolar gum loss, loosening of teeth, excessive salivation, metallic taste, tissue pigmentation, high white blood cell count (leukoplasia), low white blood cell count (leucopenia), sores in the mouth, dizziness, ringing in the ears, sensitivity to light, glaucoma, food sensitivities, colitis, diverticulitis, chronic diarrhea or chronic constipation, craving for sweets, unexplained elevated triglycerides and/or cholesterol and/or blood pressure, rapid heartbeat (tachycardia), irregular heartbeat (arrhythmia) and chest pain, repeated infections — viral and fungal — cancer, arthritis, lupus erythematosus, scleroderma, hypothyroidism, chronic headaches, allergies, dermatitis, low body temperature, clammy skin, excessive perspiration, heartburn, unexplained anemia, G6PD enzyme deficiency, chronic kidney disease, adrenal disease, loss of appetite, anorexia, nausea, ulcers, infertility, and hypoglycemia.

With a list like this, how can anyone say there is no danger because negative effects have not been seen??? So what if mercury could not be convicted in a court of law due to uncertainty in a particular case? All of these symptoms can be caused by other things. Most people have amalgam in their mouths, and most of those people have at least one, and usually more or many symptoms in the list. Even mild symptoms are undesirable. Who can say what was caused by mercury and what wasn't? Low-grade chronic mercury poisoning is difficult to detect, but impossible to reject.

If a person has complicated and varied health problems and has mercury in his teeth, his mercury levels can be estimated by measuring urinary mercury elimination, the level of mercury in a hair mineral analysis or other sophisticated testing. Even then, it is unlikely that a definite statement can be made as to what the mercury is or is not causing. Is mercury guilty or innocent? With a track record like the above list, do *you* want any of the stuff in *your* mouth? Can you allow your dentist to put it into *your child's* mouth?

"and durable"?

It is an unquestionable fact (considered unquestionable because those who question it are simply ignorant) that the mercury in amalgam is not completely stable. Vapor is constantly released into the air and the mercury dissolves into saliva. Vapor is breathed into the lungs, where approximately 80% of it is absorbed.[125] From saliva, 5-15 % is absorbed. Chewing increases the amount of vapor released for up to an hour afterward.[126] Chewing gum, anyone?

---

125   This is an average of several experimenters' estimations:
Teisinger, J. and V. Fiserova-Bergerova. 1965. *Pulmonary retention and excretion of mercury vapours in man.* Ind. Med. Surg. 34:580-584.
Neilsen-Kudsk, F. 1965. *Absorption of mercury vapour from the respiratory tract in man.* Acta.Pharmacol. Toxicol (Kbh) 23:250-262.
Hursh et al., *Clearance of mercury (Hg- 197, Hg-203) vapor inhaled by human subjects.* Archives of Environmental Health 31:302-309. 1976.
126   Vimy, M.J., and F.L. Lorscheider. 1985b. *Serial measurements of intra-oral air mercury: estimation of daily dose from dental amalgam.* Journal of Dental Research 64(8):1072-1075.

Mercury intake from amalgam is greater than the intake from eating fish and all other sources combined, including fungicides, pesticides, paints, wood preservatives, skin creams, laxatives, floor wax, wood preservatives and vaccinations. (Vaccinations may be the largest single-dose exposure; the above refers to the course of a lifetime.) Exceptions may be the unfortunate people living downwind from a coal-fired power plant, or workers in an industry which exposes them to mercury. The Mad Hatter in *Alice in Wonderland* got his nickname because hat makers were exposed to the mercury used in curing felt.

Researchers put radioactive amalgams in the teeth of sheep and followed escaped mercury with a scanner. Up the olfactory nerve went the mercury, from the nose to critical areas of the brain, such as the hippocampus, which controls memory.[127]

The fate of mercury (Hg) released from dental "silver" amalgam tooth fillings into human mouth air is uncertain. A previous report about sheep revealed uptake routes and distribution of amalgam Hg among body tissues. The present investigation demonstrates the bodily distribution of amalgam Hg in a monkey whose dentition, diet, feeding regimen, and chewing pattern closely resemble those of humans. When amalgam fillings, which normally contain 50% Hg [mercury], are made with a tracer of radioactive 203 Hg and then placed into monkey teeth, the **isotope appears in high concentration in various organs and tissues within 4 weeks.** Whole-body images of the monkey revealed that the highest levels of Hg were located in the kidney, gastrointestinal tract, and jaw. **The dental profession's advocacy of silver amalgam as a stable tooth restorative material is not supported by these findings.**[128] [Emphasis added.]

---

127 Sorry I can't give the source of this one. I found it in some old notes and cannot locate the source.
128 Hahn, et al., *Whole body imaging of the distribution of mercury released from dental fillings into monkey tissues.* Dept of Radiology, Univ of Calgary, Faculty of Medicine, Alberta, Canada FASEB J. 1991 Feb 5 (2):236. PubMed 2227216

The amount of mercury released and absorbed into bodily tissues has been found to be directly proportional to the number of amalgam fillings in the mouth. This has been consistent in too many research studies to reference here. A daily intake of 0.014 micrograms (mcg) of mercury per kilogram of body weight has been used as the "tolerable" dose, a benchmark for comparing the dose received from dental amalgam. The average weight of a 10 year-old child is 80 lbs (36 kilograms). Therefore, the "tolerable" intake of mercury each day is about 0.5 micrograms. The actual release of mercury vapor from *one* amalgam filling has been estimated by various sources at between 0.6 and 2.5 mcg, more than the "tolerable" amount. It is unclear how much of that is subsequently inhaled or swallowed and absorbed into the bloodstream, but one can easily imagine that absorption from several amalgam fillings is beyond the tolerable limit. Raised levels of mercury have consistently been found in the urine and tissues of humans and animals, depending on the number of fillings. Please note the use of the word "tolerable" in official publications and research, rather than "safe" or "acceptable." No amount is safe or acceptable.

Exposure to mercury begins in the womb. This, coupled with our knowledge that mercury exposure from new amalgam fillings quickly reaches the bloodstream and other tissues, should be enough to incriminate and, excuse me, *incarcerate* a dentist who puts mercury into the mouth of a pregnant women. The mercury from new dental amalgam has been found in maternal and fetal blood within two days. In the words of Dr. Ephraim Kahn, a California public health official, "Mercury has an affinity for the fetus and is much more toxic in unborn children than adults..."[129] This may be due to the undeveloped blood-brain barrier and means of excreting poisons from the system, as well as from the fact that mercury poisons nerve endings, which are rapidly developing in the unborn child. Exposure continues during breast-feeding:

---

129   *The New York Times*, Nov. 1, 1970

The relationship between dental history and breast milk concentration of Hg was also examined in 33 lactating women... increased Hg excretion in breast milk and urine correlated with the number of fillings or Hg vapor concentration levels in mouth air. **It was concluded that Hg originating from maternal amalgam tooth fillings transfers across the placenta to the fetus, across the mammary gland into milk ingested by the newborn, and ultimately into neonatal body tissues...**[130] [Emphasis added.]

Another disturbing study found that women with ten or more filled teeth gave birth to babies with twice as much mercury in their bodies as mothers with two or fewer amalgams.[131]

The list of mercury effects presented earlier contains numerous soul problems. We can never pin down the exact influence of mercury on our children, since there are so many other factors. However, even if we do not know exactly what it does in a particular child, we know it is bad stuff, and should be avoided to whatever extent possible in this imperfect world.

What to do?

- Instruct your dentist not to use amalgam in the mouths of your family members from this day on. There are substitute materials based on ceramics, which, although they have their problems, are not poisonous, at least to the best of our current knowledge. They also are more aesthetic, made to match the color of the teeth.
- Do not chew gum, or give your child any, if you have amalgam fillings! Chewing greatly increases the release of mercury.
- If you eat a lot of fish, check which kinds have less mercury.

---

130   Vimy MJ et al. *Mercury form maternal "silver" tooth fillings in sheep and human breast milk. A source of neonatal exposure.* Biol Trace Elem Res. 1997 Feb;56(2):143-52. PubMed 9164660.
131   My apologies again. I've lost the source!

You may consider lowering your fish consumption. If you are eating fish for the omega-3 content, you can take fish oil capsules.

- Take supplemental vitamin C (lots of it). Vitamin C may or may not remove mercury from the body (depending on whom you ask), but it changes it into less toxic forms and supports every bodily function.
- Exercise, sweat, and get plenty of fresh air.
- Eat other foods and take supplements which remove mercury:
  o Chlorella, other sea greens and algae take up toxic metals. Chlorella has been used for treating liquid industrial waste that contains metals.
  o Cilantro (coriander) — this plant is said to cause the removal of mercury and other heavy metals from the body. The scientific backing on this one is rather weak — just some anecdotal evidence — but then again, cilantro is simply a green plant that has nutritional value and a nice taste, so why not use it regularly?
  o Garlic and onion and sulfur-containing supplements — glutathione, MSM and N-acetyl cysteine. The sulfur in foods and supplements like these binds new mercury intake to prevent absorption while removing the old.
  o Selenium, the mineral, is a natural agent for chelating (grabbing like a claw) mercury. The dose is 200 to 400 mcg per day.
  o Zinc, 20 — 50 mg/day
- Removal of amalgam fillings. The health of many ill people has improved quickly after their amalgam fillings were removed and replaced. This procedure must be done by a dentist with the proper knowledge of safety procedures

and the proper equipment to minimize exposure to mercury during the process. Otherwise, the exposure could be quite heavy. For this reason, removal of amalgam fillings should not be undertaken lightly. Some dentists give intravenous vitamin C while removing amalgam fillings.

- Chelation therapy. "Chelation" is from the Greek word for claw. It describes various processes by which one substance "grabs" another. For the treatment of severe cases, a knowledgeable doctor can give chelating substances intravenously for toxic metal removal. Oral chelation products, containing a variety of beneficial substances, are available through the Internet. EDTA is a known chelator, used by conventional medicine for intravenous chelation in cases of lead poisoning. Alternative medicine doctors use it for chelating other metals, and for opening clogged arteries. Some oral products have EDTA among their ingredients. It is safe, but only 5-10% is absorbed orally. EDTA chelates some good minerals also, so its use should be followed by general mineral supplementation.

Mercury: guilty until proven innocent. And that's not going to happen.

Chapter 16

Fluoridation Farcification

Every man ... should periodically be compelled to listen to opinions which are infuriating to him. To hear nothing but what is pleasing to one is to make a pillow of the mind."
—St. John Ervine, Irish writer

Okay, I admit, "farcification" is not in the Scrabble dictionary, nor in Webster's. However, it rings true in my ears to describe the history of adding fluoride to water. What a farce! Hailed by the U.S. Department of Health and Human Services as one of the greatest health achievements of the 20th century[132], most people do not question the questionable "fact" that dumping industrial fluoride waste into the public water supply is a great idea that has vastly reduced the sugar-and-junk-food-caused rot in our children's teeth. Fluoridation is given credit for reducing tooth cavities by 40-70% from the first half of the 20th century to the second half. Fluoridation is praised as benefiting the rich and poor alike. All you have to do is drink water while you work and have your children drink water while they play. The American Dental Association loves the stuff, and has "endorsed fluoridation of community water supplies as safe and effective for preventing tooth decay for more than 40 years," because of the "overwhelming evidence of

---

132 Department of Health & Human Services Accountability Report, Fiscal Year 1999.

fluoridation's safety and efficacy."[133] The ideal medicine. No fuss, no muss. No brains either.

"No safety and no efficacy," mourns Don Quixote, his head between his hands. All the flowery statements of Don's windmills wilt in the face of a minimally objective examination of the scientific evidence.

What is fluoride?

A poisonous substance, actually, even though it is normally found in bone and teeth. Most likely, we could live without any fluoride, so intake is considered non-essential. Fluoride is fluorine, a gas, bound to another atom or molecule. It is highly absorbable through the wall of the *stomach* even at high levels — it does not even need to reach the intestine, where most dietary absorption happens. This adds to the danger, since the digestive process it avoids is a major line of defense against toxic invasion. When taken on an empty stomach, which is often done when drinking water or taking calcium fluoride tablets, or when your child swallows some of that yummy toothpaste, fluoride is 100% absorbed.[134] Milk reduces the absorption by thirty percent, so the American Society of Health-System Pharmacists recommends *not* drinking milk an hour before or after taking fluoride, whereas we think blocking fluoride absorption is a great idea. Food along with the milk may actually nullify this blocking effect[135]. In short, almost all of the fluoride we consume enters our bloodstream, gaining access to every cell. If it is safe and healthy, good; if not, bad.

Is fluoride safe?

If it is safe, why does the FDA require fluoride toothpaste to wear the

---

133   American Dental Association statement on water fluoridation efficacy and safety. June 29, 2000

134   Ekstrand J, Ehrnebo M. *Influence of milk products on fluoride bioavailability in man.* Eur J Clin Pharmacol. 1979 Sep;16(3):211-5. PubMed 499322.

135   There are several studies with different estimates of absorption with food. Most agree that food nullifies milk's affect. One study says that milk only delays, not reduces, absorption. An Indian study says that food reduces absorption greatly. All of this does not matter all that much, since fluoride is often taken alone.

label, "If you accidentally swallow more than used for brushing, seek professional help or contact a poison control center immediately"? Please put this book down and go to your tube to see for yourself.

It has long been known that too much fluoride causes irreversible tooth discoloration, which the "experts" consider to be merely cosmetic. However, this is an assumption only, and is illogical. This condition, dental fluorosis, happens to children only, meaning that it is not a su-

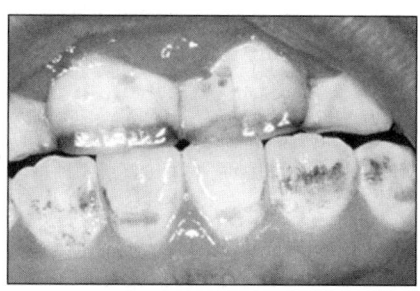

Dental Fluorosis

perficial stain or surface damage which could happen to adult teeth also, but the result of damage to the growing tooth. Fluoride damages the cells that deposit enamel, the amelocytes, causing the enamel to be porous.[136] Now I ask you, does it make sense to assume that the amelocyte is the only cell type to be damaged? Not to me. Our various cell types are more similar than they are different. There is no reason to assume that amelocytes are more vulnerable than any other.

50 Reasons to Oppose Fluoridation[137] is a well-referenced paper authored by Dr. Paul Connett, Professor of Chemistry at St. Lawrence University, New York. I will paraphrase some of the reasons he lists with a few comments of my own [in brackets]. Here we go:

40. The FDA has never approved any fluoride product for internal consumption. Drinking it is internal consumption.

41. The level of fluoride put into water is 200 times the concentration in mothers' milk.

---

136 Denbesten and Thariani. *Biological mechanisms of fluorosis and level and timing of systemic exposure to fluoride with respect to fluorosis.* Department of Biochemistry, Forsyth Dental Center, Boston, Massachusetts Journal of Dental Research, 1992 May;71(5):1238-43. PubMed 1607440.
137 *www.fluoridealert.org/50-reasons.htm*

42. Only 50% of ingested fluoride is excreted. The rest accumulates in bones, the pineal gland [reducing production of melatonin, the sleep hormone], the brain and other tissues. [Fluoride was once used to treat osteoporosis, because it really does accumulate in bone, raising bone density. However, its use for this purpose was discontinued after it was found that bone *structure* was weakened, resulting in more, not less, fractures.]

43. Fluoride causes chromosome damage and interferes with DNA repair mechanisms. [Cancer, anyone?]

44. Fluoride increased the uptake of aluminum into rats' brains. [Alzheimer's, anyone?]

45. Rats dosed before birth exhibited hyperactive behavior. [ADHD, anyone?]

46. For you chemists in the audience: fluorine is the most electronegative element. As such, it, interferes with hydrogen bonding. [Anyone knowing some chemistry and biochemistry will boggle his mind trying to imagine what *this* can cause. (Hint: for one thing, hydrogen bonds are involved in shaping protein molecules.)]

47. Fluorine slows the thyroid, and was used to treat hyperthyroidism in the early 20th century. [Fluorine is in the same atomic family as iodine, from which the thyroid gland makes its hormones. Fluorine can take the place of iodine and block thyroid hormone production. Hypothyroidism is very prevalent today, ruining the quality of life of millions. Why would that be? Hello? We are putting thyroid poison in our drinking water!!!]

48. Some people are sensitive to the fluoride concentration aimed for in drinking water, 1 ppm (part per million). This is true for healthy people, and all the more so for the elderly and the ill. [Many people suffer negative effects from drinking water with 2-3 ppm. This gives us a therapeutic index (see chapter 8) of only 2 or 3. This

is totally unacceptable in drug administration, which is what fluoridation of water *is*.

49. Fluorine was found to increase lead intake into children's brains. [Lead causes learning problems.]

50. Two hundred milligrams of the fluoride ion is enough to kill a young child. [Guess how much fluoride ion there is in a typical tube of young children's toothpaste. The answer is given below.]

51. The chemicals used to fluoridate water in many places are not pharmaceutical grade. They are wastes from the fertilizer and other industries, classified as hazardous wastes, sometimes contaminated with various impurities like arsenic. [These industries not only solved their disposal problem by dumping their hazardous wastes into our drinking supply and making us think they are doing us a favor, but they actually get paid for the stuff!]

52. At least 14 Nobel science prize winners have expressed reservations about water fluoridation.

Does fluoride prevent tooth decay?
Do we profit from facing the danger?

The sad truth is: probably not. The practice of public water fluoridation was first endorsed by the U.S. Public Health Service in 1950. There is no denying that since that time, the number of cavities in children's teeth declined radically, a fact used to manipulate the public into accepting fluoridation enthusiastically and unquestioningly, and even to take extra fluoride in tablet form, as though it were a vitamin. One chart, however, should be enough to shock the reality into anyone. Take a good look at the graph on the next page.[138]

The undeniable fact is: tooth decay dropped in all countries between 1960 and 2000, completely regardless of whether or not

---

138 This graph was prepared by Chris Neurath, Fluoride Action Network, and printed with permission. A full-color version can be found at *www.fluoridealert.org*, which has extensive writings about the fluoride issues.

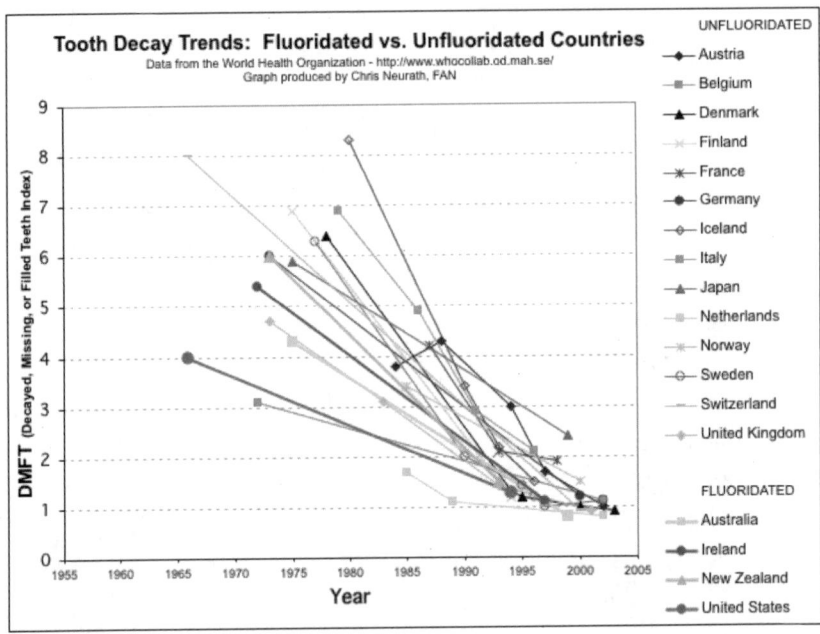

fluoride was added to the water. No one knows exactly why this occurred — perhaps because of a rise in the standard of living in most of the world, with a huge increase in the consumption of fruits and vegetables, partially due to the introduction of home refrigeration. Whatever the reason, fluoridation is hereby discredited as the Hero of Our Children's Teeth.

John Colquhoun was an early promoter of fluoridation in New Zealand, as the Principal Dental Officer in Auckland, that country's largest city. In 1997, he wrote an excellent article called *Why I Changed My Mind About Water Fluoridation.*[139] Colquhoun had become very excited about the evidence that fluoridation was improving tooth health, and, in his excitement, he overlooked evidence that tooth decay was declining equally in areas of New Zealand where the practice had not been instituted. Writes Colquhoun:

> I now realize that what my colleagues and I were doing was what the history of science shows all professionals do when their pet

---

139 © 1997 University of Chicago Press. Easily found on the Internet.

theory is confronted by disconcerting new evidence: they bend over backwards to explain away the new evidence. They try very hard to keep their theory intact — especially so, if their own professional reputations depend on maintaining that theory.

Colquhoun explains that it is impossible to find a properly conducted study. For example, in one major study, *The Hastings Fluoridation Experiment*, publicized to show fluoride's benefits, school dentists inexplicably changed their criteria for diagnosing tooth decay. Before the period of drinking fluoridated water, any small hole on the tooth was defined as decay, even before it penetrated the enamel. When the results were tallied years later, only penetration of the enamel was counted, so, of course, much less decay was found. This change was never reported in published accounts.

I do not believe that the selection and bias that occurred was deliberate. Enthusiasts for a theory can fool themselves very often, and persuade themselves and others that their activities are genuinely scientific," writes Colquhoun.

Simon and Garfunkel expressed this same idea more succinctly: "A man hears what he wants to hear and disregards the rest."[140]

Sources of fluoride other than public water

Toothpaste: There is some evidence that external application, such as brushing teeth with fluoride toothpaste, may cause a slight reduction in the number of cavities. This benefit is very much in doubt, and is outweighed by the dangers involved. Toothpaste is the most dangerous source of fluoride for children. The list above mentioned that 200 mg of the fluoride ion can kill a child. A six ounce tube of children's toothpaste typically has 0.15% fluoride ion. Six ounces rounds off to 170,100 milligrams, and 0.15% of that is 255 mg. That is how much fluoride ion is in one tube, *more than the lethal dose.*

---

140   From their song, *The Boxer.*

These toothpastes have all kinds of chemicals in them to make them tasty to children. Could you not imagine a curious child downing the whole tube? Certainly, they swallow at least a little bit with each brushing. Children have died by eating fluoride.

Here is a typical label from a popular children's toothpaste:

ACTIVE: Sodium Fluoride (0.15% w/v fluoride ion). **INACTIVES:** Water, Hydrated Silica, Sorbitol, Glycerin, Tetrapotassium Pyrophosphate, PEG-6, Disodium Pyrophosphate, Tetrasodium Pyrophosphate, Sodium Lauryl Sulfate, Flavor, Xanthan Gum, Sodium Saccharin, Carbomer 956, FD&C Blue No. 1, FD&C Yellow No. 5.
USE: Helps protect against cavities. **DIRECTIONS Adults and children 2 yrs. and older:** Brush teeth thoroughly after meals or at least twice a day or use as directed by a dentist or physician. Do not swallow. **Children under 6 yrs.:** To minimize swallowing use a pea-sized amount and supervise brushing until good habits are established. **Children under 2 yrs.:** Ask a dentist or physician.
WARNINGS: Keep out of the reach of children under 6 years of age. If you accidentally swallow more than used for brushing, seek professional help or contact a poison control center immediately.

Use this as an opportunity to practice reading product labels. Read every word. For me, even without the fluoride, it's pretty scary, with all those words I don't understand (some of them I do, and they're quite unfriendly). By the way, it would be very difficult to convince me that the "INACTIVES," all fifteen of them, are inactive — they are in the toothpaste to do something, to have chemical activity in the toothpaste. They don't stop having chemical activity after they are swallowed or absorbed through the mucous membranes of the mouth. Many authors have noted that some children ingest more fluoride from toothpaste alone than is recommended as a total daily ingestion.[141]

Processed foods and drinks: Many products contain fluoride. Instant tea, for example, has as much as 6.5 ppm, six and a half times the amount in drinking water. Infant formulas can also be a source. **"Our analysis shows that babies who are exclusively formula fed face the highest risk... more than 60 percent of the exclusively formula-fed babies exceed the safe dose of fluoride**

---

141   Levy SM, Guha-Chowdhury N. (1999). *Total fluoride intake and implications for dietary fluoride supplementation.* Journal of Public Health Dentistry 59: 211-23.

on any given day."[142] Some countries (not the U.S. or Canada) have initiated the fluoridation of salt.

Fluoride tablets: Recommended by many dentists to provide extra fluoride, they even include a bit of calcium to make them more attractive. Don't even think about it. Forget about it. It's absurd.

Teflon: Fluoride is released from Teflon pans into food, and poisonous gas is released into the air as well. Throw out your Teflon pans.

What is the moral issue?

It is immoral to force people to take medication without their "informed consent." Although some people *would* consent to fluoridation of their water supply to prevent cavities, this consent hardly can be considered "*informed*," nor should they be allowed to decide for others. When their dentist tells them to give their child fluoride tablets, they are not informed that many scientists and other informed people object to this "supplement," or that a prevalent counter-opinion says that *any* fluoride is unnecessary, useless and dangerous to the health of a child's teeth, bones, thyroid, pineal gland and everything else.

A person's response to fluoride cannot be known. Here we go again with biochemical individuality. Some people are very sensitive to even small amounts. The amount put into our water cannot be measured exactly, nor can the dose received by any particular person be controlled. On a hot day, one drinks more. So does an athlete during and after exertion. A person who drinks six 8-ounce glasses a day of water fluoridated at 1 ppm will ingest 1.5 mg of fluoride a day. Some people drink only a cup a day or less, while others drink a gallon or more. Even if some people are helped by fluoridation, others are harmed. This is immoral, and may well violate the Nuremberg Code for human experimentation.

The institutional and public support of public water fluoridation in the United States and a few other countries is unique and,

142 Environmental Working Group, *EWG Analysis of Government Data Finds Babies Over-Exposed to Fluoride in Most Major U.S. Cities*, March 22, 2006.

therefore, surprising. Fluoridation has been rejected in most countries, or outright banned by law:

Country and Fluoridation Status
- China: BANNED
- Austria: REJECTED: "toxic fluorides" NOT added
- Belgium: REJECTED: those who want fluoride should get it themselves
- Finland: STOPPED: "...do not favor or recommend fluoridation of drinking water.."
- France: "Fluoride chemicals are not included in the list [of 'chemicals for drinking water treatment']. This is due to ethical as well as medical considerations."
- Austria: "Toxic fluorides have never been added to the public water supplies in Austria."
- Germany: STOPPED
- Denmark: "... fluorides have never been added to public water"
- Norway: REJECTED: "...drinking water should not be fluoridated"
- Sweden: BANNED: No safety data available!
- Hungary: STOPPED
- Japan: REJECTED: "The regulated level is for calcium-fluoride, not the hazardous waste product which is added as artificial fluoridation."

How does this relate to the soul of my child, and what to do?
Fluoride, when ingested in excess, can have negative influences on your child's mind and emotions in several ways.

1. Dental fluorosis is unattractive and can cause lower self-image.
2. It causes increased uptake of lead — known to cause learning problems — and aluminum, a nerve poison.

3. It competes with iodine, blocking thyroid hormone production. Proper thyroid function is necessary for all of
   life's processes, including the provision of brain energy
   for learning. "Brain fog" is a symptom of hypothyroidism.
4. When it accumulates in the pineal gland, fluoride can impair production of melatonin, the sleep hormone. Sleep
   disturbances are one cause of ADHD symptoms.
5. Fluoride itself may be a cause of child hyperactivity, even
   when consumed by the mother during pregnancy.

- If you want to improve the health of your children's teeth,
  dietary improvements in the directions outlined by the 14
  Rules in Chapter 2 will be more effective than using fluo-
  ride in any form.
- If your water is fluoridated, an inverse osmosis water filter
  should get rid of it, as will activated alumina defluoridation
  filters and distillation filtration. Most other filters will not.
  Boiling the water will only concentrate the fluoride.
- Use non-fluoridated toothpaste. There are many brands.
  Choose one with the least number of ingredients you can-
  not identify.
- Avoid fluoride supplements, of course.

**Summary: Don't let those smiling, beautiful, toothy (etc.)
ladies in the commercials convince you to use fluoride toothpaste. They are getting paid for it and don't know what they
are talking about. Unfortunately, neither does your dentist, as
hard as *that* is to believe.**

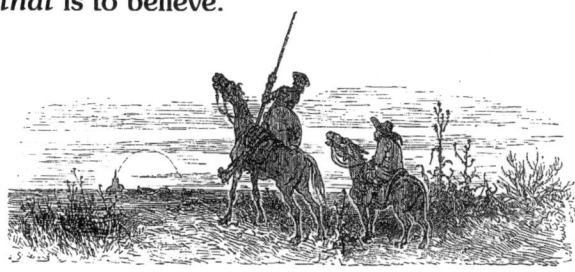

Chapter 17

ILLUSIONS !!!

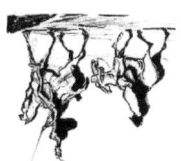

"I saw that the world is upside-down"[143]

In the sciences, people quickly come to regard as their own personal property that which they have learned and had passed on to them at the universities and academies. If someone else comes along with new ideas that contradict the Credo and in fact even threaten to overturn it, then all passions are raised against this threat and no method is left untried to suppress it. People resist it in every way possible: pretending not to have heard about it; speaking disparagingly of it, as if it were not even worth the effort of looking into the matter. And so a new truth can have a long wait before finally being accepted. — Goethe

When a windmill is unguarded, an observer may think: "Either there is nothing within to guard, or else the walls are very strong."

In my eyes, the picture that the health system chooses to present to the public — that the vaccination of children is unquestionably good — is a windmill. The walls are not strong, and any interested

---

143 From the Babylonian Talmud, spoken by one who had a near-death experience.

person can discover how they may be breached. Frightful guards are necessary, since anyone who approaches too closely will see all too clearly that the walls are a transparent illusion, and that the picture inside is not pretty. The "guards" against truth about vaccination are the one-sided approach of the medical system and the extreme emotional reaction whenever doubt is raised, accusations like "What, how can you...!!! You're endangering your children and everyone else's!!!"

I do not pretend to be an expert about vaccinations. My knowledge is based on dozens of hours of reading about the subject (an obligation for every parent), on my general knowledge of the health sciences and on my critical cynicism, born from honest examination of medical issues. While am not an expert, I rely on those who are experts in my eyes. Everyone is free to choose those they trust as experts.

I am not sure whether or not the reward-to-risk balance of vaccination is *always* negative; however, I am certain of one thing: whoever has no questions has never examined the subject at all, or is suppressing facts — intentionally or unintentionally. There are three sides to the question of vaccination and a sea of information to wade through. One side yells out "In favor!," another side cries out "Against!," and a third side says, "It depends on the particular vaccine and the particular child, and always with care." In my opinion, every parent is obliged to be aware of the various opinions about vaccinations and to make an independent decision. Every parent must take responsibility! I am a parent and grandfather who took the trouble to study the subject, in order to form an actionable opinion. Before looking into the subject, I had my children vaccinated; after studying up on it, I stopped vaccinating my youngest. I also recommend that my children not vaccinate my grandchildren.

I see no reason to present the arguments for the side that says "yes" to vaccines. That side is represented quite well by the medical establishment, from one end to the other. I rest assured that every reader has been exposed to this ~~brainwashing~~ opinion. The opposing opinion will be represented here, beginning with the words of a man who wholeheartedly believes that vaccination is poisonous, not just ineffective. Mark Sircus, founder and director of IMVA, The International Medical Veritas Association[144], wrote a book which can be downloaded for free. Its title rhymes with our own title: *Cry of the Heart: Stop Hurting Our Children.* Mark has generously allowed us to cut-and-paste a large section of the introduction to his book, which clearly describes and dismantles the first illusion about vaccines, which is:

Illusion # 1: Vaccines are responsible for the elimination of infectious disease

The Orthodoxy of Vaccines

There are many people to whom it is beyond the comprehension that there should be organized opposition to vaccines. Some of these people actually feel that a special place should be reserved in hell for people who want to kill or maim children by preventing them from receiving vaccinations, and a place in heaven should be maintained for all those who have decided it's a really good idea to inject a long list of toxic chemicals, including mercury, into little kids' bodies.

> *I felt that the first-phase results were too prone to potential biases to be the basis for important public health decisions.* — Dr. Thomas Verstraeten

Perhaps this place in hell is going to be reserved for those medical officials and scientists who have bet our children's lives on epidemiological studies that should never have been used as a basis for decisions that put our children at risk. Verstraeten is talking here about his famous study on thimerosal and autism that we will talk a lot about in this book. No matter what the truth is of the alleged

144   Website: *www.imva.info*

cover-up at the secret Simpsonwood retreat meeting[145], it is clear that huge health decisions were made on the back of flawed epidemiological studies.

This is a book about vaccines. Thus it is a book about children and what is being done to them at the hands of medical men and women. Both sides of the vaccine question are correct about one thing — lives are at stake. As such, an in-depth study of the subject is required of all parents to be. So important is vaccine study that it is a crime to deny or restrict information about it in any way. It should be required study in both high school and college. It is with this in mind that I decided to give this book away freely, so no one would be denied appropriate and easy access to this information.

The main line of the pro-vaccine side, which is repeated over and over again, is this: "Thanks to vaccines, diseases that killed or maimed millions throughout most of human history have been virtually eradicated. Where strong immunization programs exist, diseases such as polio, measles, mumps and diphtheria are scourges of the past. This remarkable achievement is periodically threatened by suspicions about vaccines that might prompt parents to resist getting their children inoculated."[146]   Medical officials fear that parents failing to vaccinate a child risk the health of the child and the larger community. They think that mass immunizations put an end to the suffering caused by rampant infectious diseases of the past. They think that the parents, who are turning their backs on the medical establishment and vaccines, have forgotten about the terrible diseases of the past that have been eradicated by vaccines.

According to the records of the Metropolitan Life Insurance Company, from 1911 to 1935 the four leading causes of childhood deaths from infectious diseases in the U.S.A. were diphtheria,

---

145 In June, 2000, fifty-two invitees from government health institutions and the major vaccine manufacturers met in the Simpsonwood Conference Center in Georgia to discuss the results of an alarming study about the effects of childhood vaccines. Although the meeting was shrouded by secrecy, it has been alleged that the main discussion of the meeting was how to cover up the negative evidence and rework the study results.
146 *USA Today* July 7, 2005 editorial

pertussis, scarlet fever, and measles. However, by 1945 the combined death rates from these causes had declined by 95%, before the implementation of mass vaccine programs.

— Harold Buttram MD

There is no actual scientific proof that vaccinations are effective and there are no control group studies, because medical authorities consider that "to not vaccinate" is unethical and have refused to study unvaccinated volunteers. What we do have is hard data collected by health officials, and the long term patterns are clear. The public has never been told that the death rate from infectious diseases fell long before vaccines were introduced, and the credit the vaccinationists insist is theirs is stolen, not earned. The entire debate that centers on benefit vs. risk ratios makes no sense when the benefits are only assumed, not proven. Immunization theory and practice are based on assumptions that do not hold water, as the chart below demonstrates:

U.S.A. DEATHS				
	Diphtheria	Pertussis	Tetanus	Measles
1901	48,839	33,094	28,065	11,956
1911	20,350	20,285	11,503	7,615
1921	12,267	14,724	7,818	4,919
1931	4,388	9,850	4,709	2,957
1941	1,135	4,399	2,384	1,013
1946	**467**	**1,460**	**1,697**	469
1951	125	558	1,093	268
1956	45	206	788	203
1961	22	82	550	**162**
1966	15	32	282	44
1971-5	12	122	122	17

[The bold numbers in shaded cells indicate the year closest to the year in which the widespread use of vaccination against each specific disease began. It is simple to see that the vaccinations had no influence on the rate of decline in the incidence of each disease. Mass vaccination against measles began in 1963. I remember that in the 1950's, our parents used to intentionally expose us to children sick with measles, chicken pox and mumps, so that we would become infected, too, and develop lifelong immunity, something that most vaccines do not provide. There actually were measles parties!]

The chart cited above is based on information found in Tim O'Shea's book, *The Sanctity of Human Blood*, and Michael Alderson's book, *International Mortality Statistics*. It shows yearly U.S. death rates for four common diseases between 1906 and 1975. The propaganda campaign for vaccination has been so successful that most of us automatically believe that vaccines are so effective they are responsible for the virtual eradication of serious childhood illnesses. Nothing could be further from the truth. "Up to 90% of the total decline between 1860-1965 in the death rate of children from whooping cough, scarlet fever, diphtheria, and measles occurred before the introduction of immunizations and antibiotics," stated Dr. Archie Kalokerinos from Australia.

The graphs below, based on the official death numbers as recorded in the Official Year Books of the Commonwealth of Australia, are taken from Greg Beattie's excellent book *Vaccination: A Parent's Dilemma* and represent the decline in death rates from infectious disease in Australia. They clearly show that vaccines had nothing to do with the decline in death rates. (Note: Graphical evidence on the decline in death rates from infectious disease for USA, England, New Zealand and many other countries shows the exact same scenario.)

Most ministries of health around the world show graphs that start in the 1950's or even 1970's to make the vaccination programs look as if they have been responsible for the eradication of diseases, but when you take the graphs back to the early 1900's or late 1800's you soon see that vaccination has done little to help the decline of said diseases. The next graphs show clearly how informa-

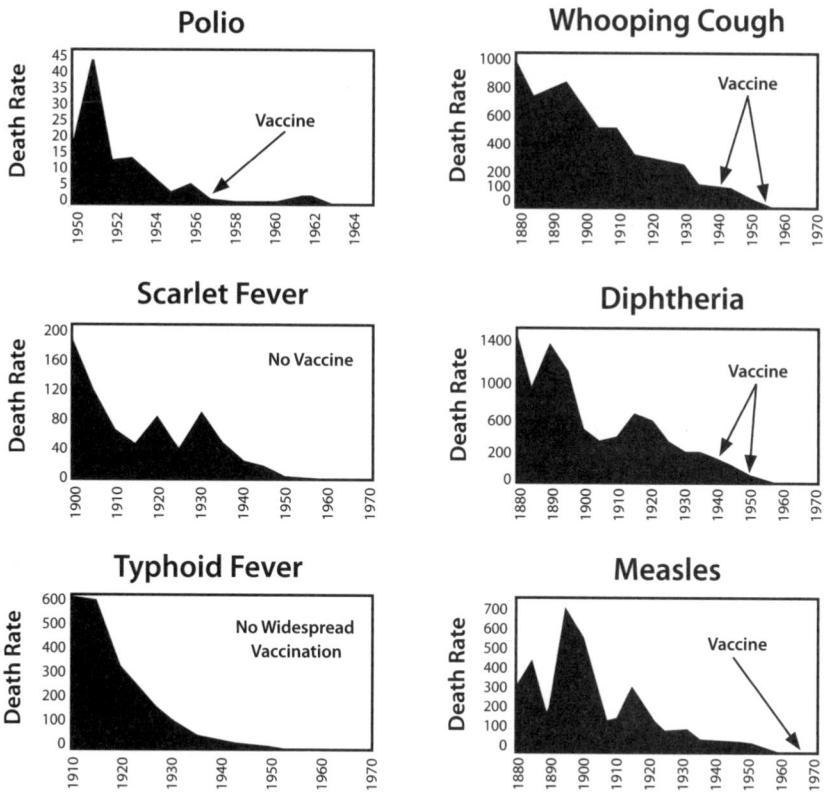

tion can be presented in an extremely misleading manner. Graph 1
leads a person to believe that the measles vaccine was responsible
for the decline of deaths, but Graph 2, which included more information going back to 1900, clearly expresses the reality that the major
part of the decline had already occurred and that the commence-
ment of vaccination had no impact on the rate of decline thereafter.

A good graph of contagious disease incidence, which begins
at 1900 (or earlier), will show a picture of death, disease incidence
and severity that declined by 90% (average) before vaccine introduction. *Plague, typhoid and scarlet fever declined without vaccine.* Measles declined in mortality 99.7% before the vaccine for it
was introduced. At some point we might inevitably conclude that
vaccine 'necessity' is a sales gimmick, not a scientific reality. Most

of the credit for the elimination of infectious diseases actually goes to better methods of sanitation, sewage disposal, and distribution of food and water.

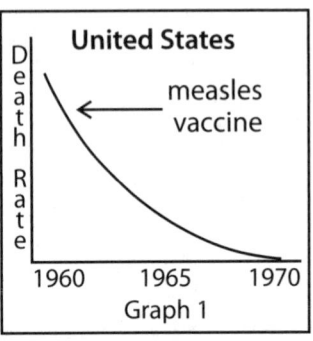

Graph 1

I'm sure that Mark Sircus will forgive me for interrupting him. The package insert for Merck & Company's measles vaccine, Attenuvax, says,

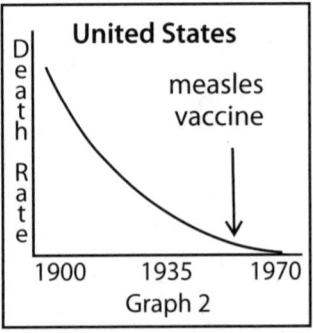

Graph 2

The impact of measles vaccination on the natural history of each disease in the United States can be quantified by comparing the maximum number of measles cases reported in a given year prior to vaccine use to the number of cases of each disease reported in 1995. A total of 894,134 cases reported in <u>1941</u> compared to 288 cases reported in <u>1995</u> resulted in a 99.97% decrease in reported cases of measles."[147]

Pay attention to the dates (underlined by me) which the company chose for comparison — 1941 and 1995. Now that Mark Sircus has educated us with the above graphs, and knowing that measles vaccines were first licensed in **1963(!)**, after a drastic reduction in measles incidence without the vaccine, (a fact which the manufacturer apparently thought would not be interesting enough to mention), we can only be appalled at the depth of the abject lies used by these people to make fools of us. When I read this, I discovered that the vaccine has a side effect of causing nausea. You don't even need to get an injection. You can get nauseous just by reading the package insert. Back to Mark (not to be confused with Merck):

---

147   *www.merck.com/product/usa/pi_circulars/a/attenuvax/attenuvax_pi.pdf*

Many of the common diseases that vaccines have been engineered to prevent show a similar graph pattern to that of polio, which today in the States only occurs from the taking of the vaccine that contains live viruses. In 1999 only eight cases of polio were reported and all were caused by the oral vaccine. Dr. Jonas Salk, developer of the first polio vaccine, testified before a Senate subcommittee that nearly all polio outbreaks since 1961 were caused by the oral polio vaccine. Salk said, "Live virus vaccines against influenza and paralytic polio, for example, may in each instance cause the disease they are intended to prevent..."[148] Dr. Sabin, developer of the newer polio vaccine, said: "Official data shows that large scale vaccination has failed to obtain any significant improvement of the diseases against which they were supposed to provide protection."[149]

Many here voice a silent view that the Salk and Sabin polio vaccine, being made of monkey kidney tissue, has been directly responsible for the major increase in leukemia in this country. — Dr. F. Klenner 150, Polio Researcher

You will never find a medical official who will debate these issues in depth. Medical authorities run from open scientific debate, for their fear is great and their assumptions weak. The vaccine question is not a religious question though it is often reduced to that by the medical press, who repeat blind beliefs because their superiors demand it. The press and the medical establishment literally prostitute themselves over the vaccine issue, keeping the public

---

148 *Science* 4/4/77 Abstracts
149 Dr. A. Sabin, developer of the Oral Polio vaccine (lecture to doctors in Piacenza, Italy, December 7, 1985)
150 Dr. Klenner was a great pioneer in the use of high doses of vitamins, particularly vitamin C. By administering vitamin C intravenously and orally, Dr. Klenner completely cured a long list of infectious diseases and other health problems. Among his incredible achievements, Klenner treated 60 children who had been diagnosed with polio. Not one of these children were left with any of the typical effects of polio, known as a crippling disease. Unfortunately (to put it mildly), Dr. Klenner's work was ignored. Vitamin C, as prevention and as cure, may have rendered the entire vaccine program unnecessary.

as confused as possible to keep vaccination rates and the profits of the pharmaceutical companies as high as possible. This book [Sircus's] looks at the realities of the immunization program and the terrible collateral damages the children are suffering from the dreadful chemicals that are put into the vaccines.

The latest furor in the vaccine area involves thimerosal, a mercury-based chemical used routinely as a preservative in childhood vaccines. Some parent activist groups claim that it causes autism, a set of developmental disorders characterized by difficulty in social interactions and behavioral problems. By the time you finish this book, you will realize that several generations of doctors and healthcare officials have been poisoning the young with mercury, using it in vaccines as a preservative without any tests to prove its safety. Such tests were impossible, for there has never been a way to prove a deadly nerve poison safe. It is the thimerosal issue that has finally cracked open shocking truths that the medical establishment and the press together have conspired to hide. The word is poison. Vaccines have contained and continue to contain poisons like mercury and aluminum that are known to cause severe neurological destruction...

The Mercury issue is not the whole issue when it comes to vaccines, but it is the issue that has already destroyed the integrity of the western medical establishment. It is the issue with the best chance of bringing medicine to its knees. It is the Armageddon of allopathic medicine and as such will be denied and covered up in much the same way any criminal denies responsibility to escape punishment and loss of image and prestige. So great is the throttle hold of the pharmaceutical companies and the medical industrialists that they have turned several generations of pediatricians into people who poison children and who feel perfectly good about it. If there were even a remotely good reason for this we might understand a little, but as this introductory chapter shows, the gains and benefits from childhood immunization is an illusion proven only in certain people's dreams.

Thank you, Mark. (For more of Mark Sircus's prolific writing and ideas, go to *www.imva.info*)

Illusion # 2: Vaccines provide immunity

The Theory of Immunity from Vaccination is very simple. We inject a weakened or dead virus or bacteria into the bloodstream. Although too weak to cause disease, this "bug" is recognized as foreign to the body, inspiring the immune system to launch an attack by millions of white blood cells. Even after the attack has destroyed the enemy, sentinels called "antibodies" are left to constantly cruise the blood, ready to repel any future attack by the same organism. In short, after the original reaction, the patient is expected to maintain lifelong immunity to the disease caused by the bug.

However much we wish it were true, this theory, as simple, as sensible and as beautiful as it is, has never been proven; in fact, many serious scientists and doctors (even non-quacks) have raised doubts. In a letter to the Congress of the United States in 1999, the scientist Vera Scheibner wrote: "There is only one immunity, and that is natural immunity, acquired through the contraction of childhood diseases." Some people have low antibody counts and are immune, while others contract a disease, despite high antibody counts.

"Not only is the pertussis vaccine only about 40 to 45% effective, but its immunity is short-lived. There is a 95% chance of infection only 12 years after vaccination."[151]

Not a cloud of doubt, however, casts its shadow on general public opinion, because most people are exposed only to vehicles of mass communication, sold out to establishment propaganda. This will end, since the truth is no longer hidden. It is available, as clear as day to any Internet user who happens upon it by chance or with the intent to learn.

It has been proven beyond a doubt that vaccines cause an immune reaction and the formation of antibodies. It is *assumed* that

---

151 Morris, J.A., *Statement Submitted to US Senate Committee on Labor and Human Relations,* June 30, 1982. (Dr. Morris served as Director of the Slow, Latent, and Temperant Virus Section of the US Bureau of Biologics, FDA).

this fact proves the effectiveness of vaccination for permanent prevention of disease; but, is this assumption correct? Here are some
simple questions for you. If the assumption is correct, why is it standard practice to give children booster shots for the same disease
they were vaccinated against previously? After a child catches the
disease, natural immunity is permanent. Why is contagion common
after vaccination? Contrary to this, scientific literature is full of proofs
that vaccines are not very effective or, even worse — there is reason
to think that they may cause more disease than they prevent. Here
are examples about various vaccines:

Polio

In 1958, there was an outbreak of polio in Israel, after vaccination
was declared mandatory and given to the majority of people. No
difference in the rate of infection was seen between the vaccinated
and unvaccinated.[152] In the Chicago Daily News (May 5, 1959), Dr.
Harold Cox from the Lederle Laboratories, one of the developers of
the Salk vaccine, was quoted as saying that the vaccine had failed
in Israel — the outbreak of polio occurred even though 90% of the
children under the age of six were vaccinated. Similar results were
found in many other countries. I personally know two men born in
1951, who contracted polio as children. One had received the vaccination, and one had not.

In the 1950's, a double-blind controlled study of the Salk vaccine
was conducted. The results were published as proof of vaccination
campaign's great success. Other researchers, however, cast serious
doubts on these conclusions, saying that the methods of gathering
data in the years following the study — including the method of diagnosis and the definition of the disease — were distorted to the extent
that it was incorrect to conclude that the vaccination was beneficial.
The opposite may be true. In 1984, Dr. Robert Mendelsohn wrote:

> For a pediatrician to attack what has become the "bread and butter"

---

152   Hearings before the Committee on Interstate and Foreign Commerce, Eighty-Seventh
Congress, Second Session on H.R. 10541, May 1962, pp.94, 96, 112

of pediatric practice is equivalent to a priest's denying the infallibility of the pope... **What is important to parents of this generation is the evidence that points to mass inoculation against polio as the cause of most remaining cases of the disease...** [My emphasis.] Meanwhile, there is an ongoing debate among the immunologists regarding the relative risks of killed virus vs. live virus vaccine. Supporters of the killed virus vaccine maintain that it is the presence of live virus organisms in the other product that is responsible for the polio cases that occasionally appear. Supporters of the live virus type argue that the killed virus vaccine offers inadequate protections and actually increases the susceptibility of those vaccinated.

This offers me a rare opportunity to be comfortably neutral. I believe that both factions are right and that use of *either* of the vaccines will increase, not diminish, the possibility that your child will contract the disease.

In short, it appears that the most effective way to protect your child from polio is to make sure that he doesn't get the vaccine! [153]

Pertussis (whooping cough)

From statistics published in the prestigious *British Medical Journal*[154], we learn that "of 8092 cases of whooping cough, 2940 were fully immunized, while only 2424 were definitely not immunized."

In Nigeria, three years after the implementation of a mass vaccination program against pertussis, a *rise* of 21% was seen in the incidence of this disease.[155]

The common side effects of the pertussis vaccine, acknowledged by *the American Medical Association*, are fever, crying bouts, a shock-like state, and local skin effects such as swelling, redness, and pain. Less frequent, but more serious side effects include convulsions and permanent brain damage resulting in mental retardation. The vaccine has also been linked to Sudden Infant Death Syndrome

---

153   Mendelsohn, R., *The Medical Time Bomb of Immunization Against Disease*, p. 52.
154   Stewart, G.T., *British Medical Journal*, January 31, 1976.
155   Ekanem, E.E., *A 10 Year Review of Morbidity from Childhood Preventable Diseases in Nigeria,* Journal of Tropical Pediatrics, Vol. 34, p. 325, December, 1988

(SIDS). In 1978-79, during an expansion of the Tennessee childhood immunization program, eight cases of SIDS were reported immediately following routine DPT immunization.[156]

Diphtheria

Official figures from the United States Army showed that the rate of death from diphtheria in the early 1980's among vaccinated soldiers was four times the rate among unvaccinated civilians.[157]

The incidence of diphtheria today is extremely low. Your child has about the same chance of being bitten by a cobra.

Measles

A measles epidemic broke out on the campus of the University of Alberta in 1987, despite a vaccination rate of 98%.[158] (See, I told you I'm not radical. I said, "despite," rather than "because of.") A comprehensive study of children in 30 states revealed that more than half of the children who became sick with measles had been properly vaccinated.[159]

Illusion # 3: Vaccines are safe

Here, my dear readers, I must apologize in advance for what I am about to tell you. Every time I study the subject of vaccine dangers, I have an anxiety attack, but I have no choice but to share my feelings with you. There are two aspects of this subject: the scientific side, needed for intellectual understanding, and the more difficult, heart-rending human side — the story of children and families whose lives turned instantly from joy to horror and sorrow.

We'll start with the scientific side. What are vaccines made of? In addition to dead or weakened viruses, there are residual

---

156 Mendelsohn, ibid.
157 Cournoyer, C., *What About Immunization? A Parent's Guide to Informed Decision Making*, Private Research Publication, Canby, Oregon, USA, 4th Edition, 1987, p. 5
158 Dayton, L., *Measles Vaccination May Not Protect for Life*, New Scientist,Vol. 4, Vancouver, Canada, November, 1989, p. 6.
159 Mendelsohn, ibid., p. 43.

proteins from the culture the viruses were grown in: pig, calf or horse blood, rabbit brain tissue, monkey or dog kidney or bird egg materials. When we eat, the proteins in our food are broken down in our digestive tracts, before they are absorbed into our blood. When proteins are injected whole, straight into the blood, bypassing digestion, they are likely to be toxic, particularly if these proteins are foreign to the human body, causing an immune system reaction. A cell biologist and researcher at the

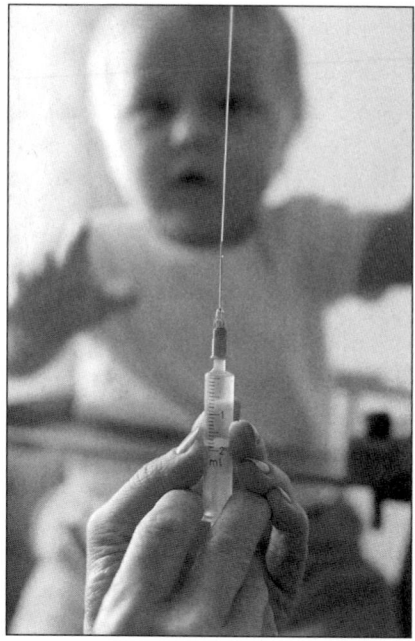

University of Wyoming, John Hoffman, wrote that vaccines "cannot help but have adverse effects on the immunologic system of the child, possibly leaving this system crippled in its ability to protect the child throughout life... opening the way for other diseases as a result of immunologic dysfunction."[160] Vital inner organs and tissues are involved in these diseases. Negative effects of vaccines are difficult to identify and may only be seen after a long time has passed.

Autoimmune diseases are those in which the immune system attacks tissues in one's own body. Due to the similarity between parts of the viruses in the vaccines and proteins in our body, such as myelin (which forms a sheath around our nerve fibers and ensures proper nerve impulse conduction), the antibodies created to defend us against the viruses may also attack the myelin and cause diseases such as multiple sclerosis and Parkinson's. Various researchers are worried that the intense schedule of vaccination imposed on infants and children can cause a list diseases later in life, including rheumatoid

---

160 Buttram, H.E., and Hoffman, J.C., *Bringing Vaccines Into Perspective*, Mothering, Vol. 34, Winter Edition,1985, p. 42

arthritis, lupus and cancer.[161] In the words of a noted Russian specialist in neurobiology, A. D. Speransky, "...it is conceivable that by these methods we may be crippling humanity."[162]

There is serious concern that immunization may be a cause of Sudden Infant Death Syndrome (SIDS). The researcher, Torch, found that two-thirds of 103 infants who died of SIDS had been given the triple diphtheria-pertussis-tetanus (DPT) vaccine less than three weeks before their death, and many of them died within 24 hours of the injection.[163] In a publicized incident in Tennessee, eleven babies died within eight days of the DPT vaccination, eight of them within 24 hours.[164] **Vaccines are killing babies.**

In September 1997, more than 500 doctors, scientists, health officials and legal experts from five countries convened for the First International Public Conference on Vaccination. Among the opinions and observations that the various speakers presented were[165]:

- The pertussis vaccine is particularly toxic to the human brain and should be immediately withdrawn from the market.
- The triple DPT vaccine, which can cause brain inflammation and severe brain damage, is also capable of causing minor forms of brain damage, such as learning disabilities and ADHD.
- Live viruses, such as those used in the MMR vaccine (measles, mumps, rubella), which is now linked to autism, have

---

161   Dettman, G., *Immunization, Ascorbate and Death*, Australian Nurses Journal, December, 1977.

162   *Immunization Public Health Protector?*, Issued under NIB National Office of Health Development, Ottawa, Canada, 1979, p. 8

163   Torch, W., *Diptheria-Pertussis-Tetanus (DPT) Immunization: A Potential Cause of the Sudden Infant Death Syndrome (SIDS)*, Neurology, No. 32, 1982, p. A169

164   Mortimer, E., Jr., *Pertussis Immunization: Problems, Perspectives, Prospects*, Hospital Practice, October, 1980, pp. 103-118

165   Dr. Raymond Obomsawin, *Immunization: Medical Miracle or Masterful Mirage*, pp. 8-9. Information on the conference is available from: National Vaccine Information Center: #206-512 W. Maple Avenue, Vienna, VA, USA, 22180, Telephone: 1-800-909-SHOT

never been investigated for their long-term immune and neurological effects, and may cause genetic damage.

- Many adults have suffered central nervous system damage or death after being injected with the hepatitis B vaccine. *This vaccine is routinely injected into babies in the first hour after birth.*
- Polio vaccines contaminated with monkey viruses are a suspected cause of the development of HIV and some rare cancers.
- Data from New Zealand and other countries suggests that early vaccination has caused an increase in juvenile diabetes.
- Government health officials have withheld information about vaccines from the public.

The consensus among research scientists who attended was that current immunization programs are causing injuries and deaths because of inadequate vaccine safety research, testing, manufacturing and monitoring for long term effects.

In addition to the viruses in vaccines, please note that most preparations also contain assistants, or "adjuvants," and preservatives, such as:

- Formaldehyde — a preservative that we all became acquainted with in our school science classes. We embalmed insects in it.
- Mercury — a known neurotoxin
- Aluminum — also a nerve poison, suspected of causing Alzheimer's (in the lineup with mercury) and other disorders
- Acetone — an inflammable substance, used in nail polish remover
- Phenol (carbolic acid) — a poisonous substance, particularly caustic.

These nice additives kick the immune system into overdrive to activate the vaccination process. Unfortunately, this overstimulation can cause the immune system to attack unintended targets, similar to "collateral damage," the killing of civilians in a war. We do not know the exact fate and influence of these materials in our children's bodies, but we

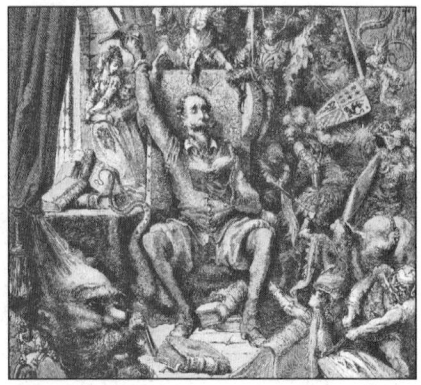

Don Quixote speaks of Vaccination

can be pretty sure that they are not vitamins. I find it slightly difficult to accept that these materials are being injected into the pure bloodstreams of my children and grandchildren, *or into yours.* The "informed consent" required by law before a medical procedure is ignored in the case of vaccines. Now you are being informed.

From the halls of the FDA, the American Food and Drug administration, came a joy-bringing announcement in 2000: "Vaccines contain safe amounts of mercury." Wonderful!!! Finally I was able to sleep in peace, until I learned that on the day he is born, a child may have 12.5 milligrams of mercury injected straight into his bloodstream, in some of the vaccines against hepatitis B. I took out my pocket calculator and figured out that this is 35 times the "permitted" daily intake of mercury.[166] Since 1940, the number of required doses has risen to 40 doses of 12 different vaccines. An infant may receive up to 62.4 micrograms of mercury in one visit. Even worse, the "permitted" amount is for an adult, not a baby, in whom there are at least three physiological differences that make the mercury injection even more dangerous:

1. A baby has not yet developed his blood-brain barrier and,

---

166   According to the Environmental Protection Agency, the safe amount of mercury is 0.1 microgram for every kilogram of body weight (Journal of the American Medical Association, 1999). If so, a baby weighing 7.7 pounds (3.5 kilograms) can handle 0.35 micrograms of mercury.

therefore, mercury flows freely into the brain tissue. The form of mercury in vaccines has a particular attraction to nerve cells, so the mercury can lodge in the infant's brain until after the blood-brain barrier forms, trapping it inside.

2. A baby does not yet manufacture liver bile, needed to carry mercury out of the body.

3. The "permitted" amount is for oral intake. Any absorption limitation is bypassed by injection straight into the blood!

A few words are in order here about immediate reactions to vaccination shots. About 3,300,000 children are vaccinated every year in the United States. Around 16,000 of them, one out of 200 or so, react with extended, high-pitched screaming for several hours after the shot. Many neurologists consider this a manifestation of central nervous system over-stimulation. Hello? Vaccination is intended to stimulate the *immune system*, not the *brain*! In addition to those who simply scream, about 8,500 children suffer convulsions, and a similar number collapse in a state of shock. Not bad odds, if you figure it out statistically. "A small price to pay for the elimination of disease," you may say, if you live inside a windmill. Oh yeah, and if it's not *your* statistically insignificant child.

Do vaccines cause autism, like the vaccine-deniers claim?

We certainly had better not depend on the medical establishment to give us an honest answer to this one. Can you imagine the American Medical Association admitting: "Yes, we destroyed the lives of millions of children and parents and caused untold suffering by ignoring all negative evidence. Sorry about that, folks. Every day, in every way, we are getting better and better."? Ain't gonna happen. That would cost too much money in lost class action suits.

What sort of proof is needed? Again, innocent until proven guilty? Would we let a suspected rapist-murderer run wild in the streets, until proof of guilt is established in a court of law? When it comes to a simple vitamin, before its use is recommended or even allowed for the treatment of a particular disease, clear and outstanding proof of benefit is demanded, while it must never, but *never*, cause any unpleasantness, even so much as gas in the belly. Juxtaposed to this, the mercy and forgiveness displayed by windmill dwellers towards the side effects and toxicity of vaccines scream to the high heavens, in extended, high-pitched screaming.

Autism is a true epidemic. Statistics from the United States teach us that the number of children stricken by autism grew from one child out of 10,000 in 1978, to one child among 150 in 2004, totaling 500,000 children!!!!! The establishment has not found a cause. No one has found a complete cure. They say that autism is a genetic problem, a diagnosis that removes guilt from everyone and everything. This is impossible, however; an epidemic can not be a genetic problem. Epidemics spread very quickly, while genes change very slowly. There most certainly is a genetic susceptibility to problems caused by environmental factors, but the environmental factors must be the major cause, while the genetics is only secondary. Bernard Rimland, a renowned autism researcher, said in an interview:

> My autism book, "Infantile Autism," which was published in 1964, established beyond any doubt that there is a strong genetic element in autism. In the present instance, the genetic element seems, on the basis of a good deal of evidence, that the children have a tremendously difficult time detoxifying heavy metals, including mercury. There are differences of 10,000 percent in the sensitivity of some individuals vs. others in their sensitivity to mercury. Many of the vaccines that these autistic kids have been given contain huge amounts, very, incredibly large amounts of extremely toxic mercury, which was put in there as a preservative.

Scientists are restricted in their declarations by professional etiquette and accepted criteria of proof. Not so quacks like us, the budding knights of Don Quixote, free to express the cries of our hearts, according to what our intense research, intuition and life experience has revealed to us, and those that hear may accept or reject our opinions. And therefore we declare:

VACCINATION IS A CAUSE OF AUTISM!

Scientific "proof," if, according to the philosophy of science, there truly is such a thing as proof, has several components. First, rationale: it must make sense. Mercury is a nerve poison, a fact that no one denies. A person does not have to be a genius, a scientist or a knight to conceive of a connection between a nerve poison and poisoning nerves. The most important part of the brain is nerve cells, which enable us to think, communicate and act normally. A long list of symptoms is common to mercury poisoning and autism. "We have shown that every major characteristic of autism has been exhibited in at least several cases of documented mercury poisoning."[167]

The next candidates for election as causes of autism are the active ingredients in vaccines, especially the triple vaccine for measles-mumps-rubella (MMR), even without mercury. The MMR was added to the list of mandatory vaccines in 1978 (which so happens to be the year mentioned above as the starting point for the rise-of-autism-in-the-United States statistics).

A disruption of the proper functioning of the intestine is common in autistic children. In 1996, Dr. Andrew Wakefield, a gastroenterologist and surgeon in London, began to examine the intestines of autistic children. He discovered a new pathology: lymphoid nodular hyperplasia[168], or, for us simple humans, the swelling of lymph nodes in the intestines. The body interprets the resulting lump as something that must be expelled, and the intestine contracts to expel it.

---

167 Bernard and others, *Autism: a Novel Form of Mercury Poisoning*. Published on the website of the Autism Research Institute at the link: *www.autism.com/triggers/vaccine/mercury.htm*. A fully referenced chart comparing the two is found in the article.

168 Wakefield, et.al. *The significance of ileo-colonic lymphoid nodular hyperplasia in children with autistic spectrum disorder*. European Journal of Gastroenterology and Hepatology, vol 17 #8.

Unfortunately, the lump is attached to the intestinal lining, and so the intestine folds up like parts of a telescope. Wakefield also discovered that the accompanying intestinal inflammation is an autoimmune reaction (the immune system is attacking body tissue as though it were a foreigner). What can cause the intestine of a two-year-old child to be attacked as if it were a foreign body? Wakefield, partnering with Professor John O'Leary, an expert in molecular biology, found the measles virus in the intestine of almost every autistic child. The two researchers identified beyond a doubt that the source of the virus was the measles component of the MMR.[169] Wakefield is continuing his work, despite the intense opposition of the establishment, which refuses to fund his research and has made every effort to besmirch his name. Wakefield's conclusion is that there is a high probability that the MMR triple vaccine is a cause of autism.

After establishing rationality in the process of proving something scientifically, we turn to population studies, or "epidemiology," in scientific jargon. The Amish populations in Ohio and Pennsylvania live according to traditional ideals — religion, family, manual labor and simplicity. They work the land by horse or oxen-drawn plows, avoid modern excesses — and have rejected vaccinations. According to government statistics, in the general population, an average of one out of 166 children are stricken by autism; however, among the Amish in the area of Middlefield, Ohio, only one out of their 15,000 children is autistic. This child was vaccinated. This finding is typical among the Amish in other areas.

"In China, where the disease was virtually unknown prior to the introduction of thimerosal by U.S. drug manufacturers in 1999, news reports indicate that there are now more than 1.8 million autistics," wrote Robert F. Kennedy, the most famous warrior against the use of mercury in vaccines. Although the FDA has removed thimerosal from many vaccines in the United States, the offending companies have been allowed to export it to other countries. This, of course, will not be considered honorable foreign policy when the ramifica-

---

169   O'Shea, Tim. *The Sanctity of Human Blood*. Two Trees; 8th edition (June, 2004)

tions are worked out. Kennedy's article, revealing the extent of cover-ups, bribery and conflicts of interest surrounding the revelation that vaccines are causing horrible health problems, appeared in *Rolling Stone Magazine* on June 20, 2005. It is recommended reading, and available on the Web.

The windmills also use epidemiological (population) studies to show the opposite, that vaccines are safe and effective. However, many questions have been raised about the design and statistical interpretation of these studies, and doubt has been cast on the truth of their conclusions. The studies have been interpreted as indicating that there is no proof that vaccination is connected to autism; however, what is *not* stated is that the studies also do not prove that there is *no* connection. Epidemiology has been called "a blunt tool" and can rarely be used as the major factor in policy formation. It is open to bias and can be used to prove anything. In this case, epidemiology has been used as a hired gun. The campaign against Wakefield and other researchers and parents who dare to question vaccine safety is based on several epidemiological studies. *In none of these studies were the parents of autistic children interviewed and questioned about their experiences, nor was a single child examined!!!*

In the eyes of any good, conservative scientist, a personal story, whether told by a layman or a doctor, has close to zero value as scientific proof. Neither does a group of such stories. This is called "anecdotal" evidence, which can only be used, if at all, to suggest lines of future research. Sometimes this approach is ridiculous. According to this approach, it has never been proven that a person will die if he jumps out of an airplane without a parachute. In some cases, ignoring anecdotal reports is illegitimate, even if taking them seriously costs someone power and money. Since the scientific method belittles anecdotal reports, no matter how numerous, We The People must vote with our feet, not waiting for "proof." Thousands of parents have dutifully brought their children to their loving pediatrician for vaccination, and then watched in unimaginable horror while their children began the tumble towards autistic hell within a day. "They will forever remain convinced that vaccines were responsible for the drastic changes their previously normal and healthy children exhibited post-MMR. Their stories are shockingly similar: A child, four times to one a boy, who is developmentally, socially and verbally on par for his age, suddenly stops acquiring new words and skills after his MMR vaccination, and then regresses into the abyss of autism, losing speech, cognitive abilities and social dexterity."[170] These parents have witnessed this and told about it. No parent would lie about this. We believe them.

On the other side is the Center for Disease Control (CDC) of the Department of Health and Human Services, which gives unreserved support for all vaccination policies. One might think that they live in a different world, or in a soundproof windmill. What they have to say about the autism and vaccine connection is:

- Because signs of autism may appear at around the same time children receive the MMR vaccine, some parents may worry that the vaccine causes autism.
- Carefully performed scientific studies have found no relationship between MMR vaccine and autism...
- Groups of experts, including the American Academy of Pediatrics, agree that MMR vaccine is not responsible for recent increases in the number of children with autism. In 2004, a report by the Institute of Medicine (IOM) concluded that there is no association between autism and MMR vaccine, or vaccines that contain thimerosal as a preservative.

And in the words of Dave Tayloe Jr., MD, President of the American Academy of Pediatrics (AAP):

It is important for families to trust their pediatricians instead of those who believe, with no scientific evidence [sic], that vaccines cause more harm than good. If the anti-vaccine trend continues

170   Yazbak, *MMR and Autism*, 2002.

to grow, we will surely have measles, mumps and whooping cough epidemics in our communities, and we will add to the one-quarter million deaths that occur from measles each year in developing countries without access to vaccines. The United Kingdom has already declared measles to be endemic there.

There must be something wrong with my brain, because both sides seem so *believable*. Perhaps this is a right brain/left brain kind of disorder, like a lobotomic severing of the connection, which makes it impossible to reconcile two opinions. Maybe a psychiatrist reading this can explain to me how two diametrically opposed views can exist in one world. Am I schizophrenic? My mind jumps back and forth, according to what I'm reading at the moment. The CDC reassures me with their studies, but when I read parental reports, such as the following, I think that these parents must be so deeply insulted by the CDC's reassurances that someone should be sent to prison for public defamation. Here is a typical story:

Hello,

I am the mother of two children who were damaged by vaccines. The first is autistic! No, he was not born that way. He was completely fine until the age of nine months. Then he had a very severe reaction to vaccination. He developed convulsions, lost his verbal ability and lost communications with his surroundings and rapidly deteriorated. His care now costs thousands of dollars a month.

We waited until the second child was one year old, and then gave him "only" the diphtheria-tetanus shot, because we felt the tetanus was important. After the vaccination he regressed from walking to crawling and from solid food back to liquid. He was almost completely unable to eat and did not stop vomiting. His temperature rose very high, and he became jaundiced with no signs of a virus. Blood tests showed values for liver enzymes like those of hepatitis... The doctor did not believe that this was connected to the vaccination. His health continues to deteriorate...

We must not put our heads in the sand. Our children are being poisoned, and those responsible are, at best, whitewashing information they prefer we should not know. At worst, they are lying. This is my personal conclusion, from which I cannot hide. The public is supposed to depend on the windmill giants 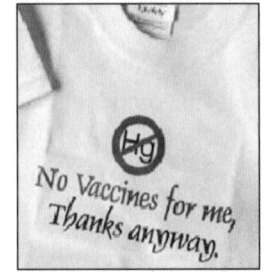 of the modern medical system to conduct their affairs honestly, placing public good above all and keeping us informed. Don't count on it. Offering honest information would remove the army that guards the windmill, allowing access to see what is inside. Fortunately, access to all necessary information is freely available on the Internet. We must learn to depend on ourselves, not on the windmills; they have their own, mixed interests in mind.

When taking responsibility for forming an educated and actionable opinion about vaccines, everyone will experience the seesaw of being influenced by whatever he or she is reading at the moment. This is the way of the world — knowledge is hard to come by. The only way to come to a conclusion is to continue studying both sides, until, at some point, one of the sides ceases to convince. I am no longer on the seesaw.

An Alternate View of the Causes of Infectious Disease

> "The devil take thee for a clown," said Don Quixote "and what shrewd things thou sayest at times! One would think thou hadst studied."

> "Human beings, the potentially highest form of life expression on this planet, have built the vast pharmaceutical industry for the central purpose of poisoning the lowest form of life on the planet--germs! One of the biggest tragedies of human civilization is the precedence of chemicals over nutrition."
> — Dr. Richard Murray

Following even the most horrible plagues that ever visited mankind, some people stayed alive. This does not need to be proven, for behold, I am here writing, and you are here reading. When flu strikes in a school, the rate of student absence may reach a third, while two-thirds remain healthy, although exposed to the same virus. We live in a world swarming with pathogens, disease-causing organisms, to which everyone is exposed every day, and yet we remain generally healthy. Right now, there may be 50,000 or a million bacteria on each square inch of your skin.

Bacteria and other microbes — germs — are part of the major cycles of nature. For them, the world is a huge garbage processing and recycling factory. If these little things were non-existent, every single animal that ever died would be lying around dead and whole, and no plant material would rot and feed the forest floor. Life would be impossible. Love Thy Germs.

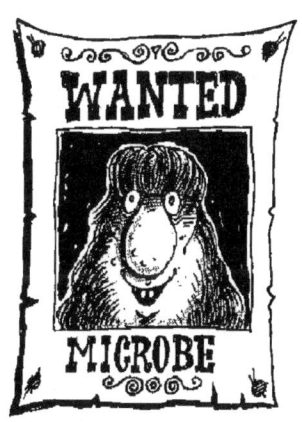

These critters have the same job in a human body that they have elsewhere in nature. They are scavengers, cleaning up what needs to be cleaned up, breaking down waste. In humans, they aid digestion and even create some nutrients as byproducts. Our bodies are densely populated with microorganisms, inside and out. They do not hurt us; rather, they are essential. They are more numerous than cells. (We are each made of around 60 trillion cells.) We live with them in a mutually beneficial relationship. *They do not attack live, healthy cells.* They scavenge diseased, malnourished tissue and multiply as they feed on it. *They are no more responsible for disease than maggots are responsible for garbage.*

A battle existed among the great scientists of the past, and it continues today. It is a battle of minds, knowledge and understanding, manifesting itself as the choices made to prevent and treat disease. Does a microbe cause a disease by uninvited attack (the germ theory), or is the disease a side effect of the microbe's natural life-cycle, as it lives on diseased terrain (the terrain theory)? Although Louis Pasteur has been popularized as the father of the germ theory of disease, his work was predated by Rudolf Virchow, who said, in his last days:

> If I could live my life over again, I would devote it to proving that germs seek their natural habitat—diseased tissue—rather than being the cause of the diseased tissue; mosquitoes seek the stagnant water, but do not cause the pool to become stagnant.

Even Pasteur, on his death bed, was reported as saying, "It's the terrain, not the germ." Nonetheless, germ theory has lived on, and has been embraced by one of the most profitable business interests humankind has ever seen, supported by a global infrastructure. It has enabled drug companies to target specific "enemies," developing research institutes and medical study programs to promote the international use of their products. A large chunk of the resulting profits has been used to brainwash the public, to the extent that drugs are the first thing most people reach for to solve all health and soul problems. The war against microbes has indeed saved lives, because the symptoms of disease are controlled by the massacre of microbes, but the underlying basis of the disease is ignored and festers. This works out just fine for the drug companies and the medical-industrial complex enslaved to them. The underlying weakness of the tissues — of human biochemistry, physiology and metabolism — which invites disease, remains, and the drug companies will sell green and red pills to treat the side effects of their purple and yellow ones, creating a worldwide addiction to their profitable wares. Pasteur's nemesis, who supported the terrain theory, Antoine Bechamp, said, "There is no doctrine so false that it does not contain some particle of truth."

Do we need to build defenses or create health?
In 1914, Rosenow showed that bacteria change their forms according to the medium in which they are grown. After changing the

content of the medium, he was able to watch pathogenic bacterial forms become benign forms, and then reverse back to pathogenic when the original medium was restored! Changes of this type could take place within two days. Disease, he concluded, was not dependent upon the microbes existing in the environment, but on what happens to them inside us! Various other scientists came to similar conclusions, notably Rife: "We are of the opinion that if the body's metabolism was kept in perfect balance... the body would be impenetrable to disease."[171]

Further proof of this line of thinking came from the work of Alexis Carrel at the Rockefeller Institute. Carrel infected mice, fed an accepted lab mouse diet, with an infectious disease, and 52% of them died. When he improved the diet step-by-step in succeeding groups, the death rate dropped, first to 32%, then to 14% and, on a very enriched diet, none died![172]

The established medical system looks to unravel the mystery of disease in a test tube, but the true place to look is on our dining room tables. If your child has sugared cereal for breakfast every morning, followed by a pastrami sandwich on white bread for lunch and pizza for dinner, with junk food snacks in between, and cola or other sweet drinks are his liquid nourishment, his metabolism will be unbalanced and he will have multiple nutritional deficiencies. His terrain will be friendly to "disease-causing" microbes. Maybe he does need vaccines then, but maybe not, because a weak body is also susceptible to the side effects of vaccines. It is possible that attacking microbes is more appropriate when the body is weak, offering disease organisms a home. The doctor must then make war against the little critters with drugs, which pollute the body and weaken it even more, instead of strengthening it naturally, the way good food does.

Creating health is the best way to defend against the organisms of disease: learning and applying the message of Dr. Weston Price,

---

171 Seidel, R.E., and Winter, E., *The New Microscopes*, Journal of the Franklin Institute, Vol. 237, No. 2, February, 1944, pp. 103-130
172 Carrel, A., *Man the Unknown*, Harper Brothers, New York and London, 1935, p. 7

choosing good, whole foods, adding vitamins and minerals, drinking water and the natural juices of fruits and vegetables, avoiding bad habits and getting physical exercise. In short, living in harmony with nature as much as possible, according to the Fourteen Rules set out in the second chapter of this book.

For disease prevention, of special concern is a high daily intake of vitamin C. Seventy years of clinical observation and thousands of studies have shown that this vitamin prevents and cures infectious disease.[173] Whoever has the gall to deny this does not know what he is talking about, whether or not he has capital letters after his name. Even many who are dedicated to natural medicine speak against giving effective doses of vitamin C, based on superficial knowledge or philosophy. Every physical or mental stress drains the body of vitamin C, and without it, our immune system is weakened, paving the way for pathogens. Vitamin C treatment is simple, cheap and available to all, and therefore unattractive to anyone who has spent years studying conventional or natural medicine. This is another subject where the responsibility rests on parents. Go and study. Search the Internet for "orthomolecular" and "vitamin C," and spend a few hours reading[174]. Long before you finish, you will know far more than 99% of doctors and 80% of naturopaths and nutritionists about guarding your health with vitamin C.

Another vitamin vital to proper immune system functioning is Vitamin "L." It is known that LOVE releases endorphins, those world famous feel-good substances. Dr. Candice Pert, researcher and author of the groundbreaking book, *The Molecules of Emotion*, taught us that viruses enter cells using the same receptors used by endorphins. There is competition between the two. Give your child the Vitamin L Advantage, to power natural immunization.

---

173   The best, most complete source of information on this subject is Dr. Thomas Levy's book, *Vitamin C, Infectious Diseases, & Toxins: Curing the Incurable*. The book has over 1200 scientific references.

174   The best places to start your studies of vitamin C may be, *www.vitamincfoundation.org*, and *www.doctoryourself.com*. On these sites and the links provided, you can find enough information to keep yourself occupied for years, during which your health will improve considerably.

In summary, if your child has an immune system fed by proper nutrition, the odds are that she will not be among those infected with microbial disease, or even the common cold. And if her resistance breaks down, act immediately: give your child as much vitamin C as she can tolerate, exactly as recommended by the vitamin C charlatans, the students of Don Quixote, those who see what millions are blind to.

If, after all, you decide to give your children all or some of the vaccines

You can offer them some protection against bad reactions by giving them vitamin C. The Australian physician, Dr Archie Kalokerinos, says:

> If the Vitamin C status of an infant is borderline, the administration of a vaccine, particularly (but not only) pertussis vaccine, can result in endotoxemia. This results in a severe reaction to the vaccine, a tremendous increase in the need for Vitamin C, and the precipitation of some of the signs and/or symptoms of acute scurvy. The onset of this may be so rapid that the classical signs of scurvy may be absent. Sudden death, sudden unconsciousness, sudden shock or sudden spontaneous bruising and hemorrhage (including brain and retinal hemorrhages) may occur. Hemorrhage and bruising in such cases can be wrongly attributed to the 'battered baby syndrome'.[175]

The great Dr. Abram Hoffer advised parents to give their child *at least* one gram of vitamin C before vaccination.[176] Even better would be to give vitamin C every day of your child's life (and take it yourself every day of yours), increasing the amount several days before and after vaccination. The addition of a multivitamin is also an excellent idea.

---

175   Kalokerinos, Archie. *Every Second Child.* Keats Publishing, 1981.
176   Hoffer, Abram. *Dr. Hoffer's ABC of Natural Nutrition for Children.* Quarry Health Books (2001) p.159.

If you decide to vaccinate your child, there are other precautions you can take. Many believe that it is advisable to delay some or all vaccinations until the child is a bit older. The routine inoculation of newborns with the Hepatitis B vaccine is particularly unjustified, unless a mother has hepatitis B, or if you expect your baby to hang out in bars, inject street drugs and engage in promiscuous sex before the age of one year. Any other newborn simply does not need it so early. This vaccine is given to every baby because of these rare cases. The only ones profiting from this program are... well, you know who.

In Japan, between 1970 and 1974, the DPT vaccine was administered between the ages of 3 to 5 months old. The Japanese health care system made damage payments for 37 deaths and 57 cases of permanent disability caused by this vaccination. From 1975 to 1980, the vaccine was given at two years of age, and only eight serious reactions, including three deaths, were recorded, a reduction of 90%.

There has never been an authoritative study done to check the safety of mixing more than one vaccine in a vial. Triple vaccines (or even quintuple) are given for convenience only. Triple vaccines contain more dangerous additives, and they stress the child's immune system to a greater degree, perhaps synergistically. Single-dose vaccines do exist, and it is possible and desirable for parents who decide to vaccinate their children to demand that only one vaccine be given at each visit to the doctor.

Some have expressed concern when reading this information, because they feel powerless. Schools have forbidden entry to unvaccinated children, and social workers have threatened to have children torn from their "irresponsible" parents. There are legal options available for parents in trouble to declare their opposition to vaccination on moral and religious grounds, since freedom of religion is guaranteed by the First Amendment. Please refer to Dr. Andrew Saul's website, *www.doctoryourself.com*, for preliminary information, and go on from there.

We will conclude this chapter as we began, by quoting Mark Sircus:

The increase in the amounts of vaccines being developed and implemented for everything under the sun should be a red flag for any parent.

It is a difficult situation because parents depend on their pediatrician's advice and counsel in their decision to vaccinate their children. Standing one's ground on medical issues in the face of one's doctors and the entire medical establishment position is not easy, but that is exactly what parents need to do. Parents must learn more than the doctors, who have their AMA and APA blinders on. It is actually very hard though, to stand your ground in front of most doctors, who consider themselves the be all end all of medicine and medical treatment. True medical wisdom begins when we become aware of what we do not know, but this is sorely absent today in modern medicine.

Doctors look at you like you are crazy when you refuse something they think you should try. They are dumbfounded when you let them know what the reasons are for our refusal of vaccines and toxic medicines, even when we explain that we have seen the studies, the information that is hidden or downplayed by public health officials.

If the pediatricians would at least become more responsible about when they vaccinate, how they vaccinate and whom they vaccinate, it would help the cause of their integrity a lot. Most pediatricians vaccinate without paying attention to the contraindications. They shoot the kids up with many vaccines even when a child's immune system is compromised, even when strong nutritional deficiencies or illnesses are present. Many pediatricians seem to have forgotten that "First Do No Harm" to the children is their obligatory vow.[177]

Well, dear readers, this chapter on vaccinations is certainly not complete, but is now ended, except for a few comments below, first by Albert Einstein, and then by your humble author.

---

177   Sircus, Mark. *Doctors & No-Vaccine Families*. Oct. 2005. *(www.thenhf.com/vaccinations_69.htm)*

Only two things are infinite: the Universe and human stupidity, and I'm not certain about the former.

—Albert Einstein

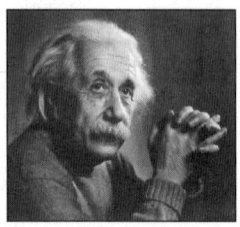

Some personal comments on this chapter:

1. No one should let me or anyone else tell them what to do about vaccines. The responsibility for decisions in child-raising is the parents', not their doctor's, and certainly not the government's. I am against governmental interference in decision-making processes in most issues. The responsibility is the parents', because they must live with the results and, even more so, because they are the ones whose *love* is the sole incentive lighting their path.

2. There is a massive amount of information out there, so the mandatory task of self-education is not easy. Eventually, however, a person's path will become clear.

3. A battle of statistics can be endlessly fought, each side bringing in the troops of studies to support his position. Everyone sees what they want to see, even yours truly. There's no vaccination against personal bias.

4. In making decisions about vaccinations, it is advisable to take into consideration the dangers and benefits of each disease and each vaccine, and to consider the individual health and strength of the child involved.

5. In 1988, in response to the growing public pressure and rising pile of evidence, the FDA "recommended" that the drug companies remove thimerosal from their vaccines. Since then, thimerosal has been removed from many, but not all, vaccines. The remaining inventory, however, was not removed from the shelves, but marketed. I have no idea what remains today. Some say they tested vaccines and found mercury, even though it is not listed as an

ingredient. Some say that thimerosal is used in vaccines that are exported to children far away. After all, *they* are not *our* problem. All of the warnings about other substances in vaccines are still valid.

6. Finally, I have made a tremendous effort to be accurate; however, with the millions of pages of information available about vaccines, it is impossible to examine every quote and every sentence in proper depth. I have one final thing to say in my defense: if a few inaccuracies are uncovered in this chapter, or anywhere in this book, for that matter, and if my viewpoint is not completely balanced, ***it's sure a hell of a lot more accurate and balanced than the info ground up and spewed out by the medical authority windmill.***

"Hold your peace, my daughters," said Don Quixote; "I know very well what my duty is; help me to bed, for I don't feel very well; and rest assured that, knight-errant now or wandering shepherd to be, I shall never fail to have a care for your interests, as you will see in the end." And the good wenches (for that they undoubtedly were), the housekeeper and niece, helped him to bed, where they gave him something to eat and made him as comfortable as possible.

At this point, my friends, this book, too, must end, for it can never be completed.

"Acquire the courage to believe in yourself. Many of the things that you have been taught were at one time the radical ideas of individuals who had the courage to believe what their own hearts and minds told them was true, rather than accept the common beliefs of their day."
     — Unnamed apprentice of Don Quixote

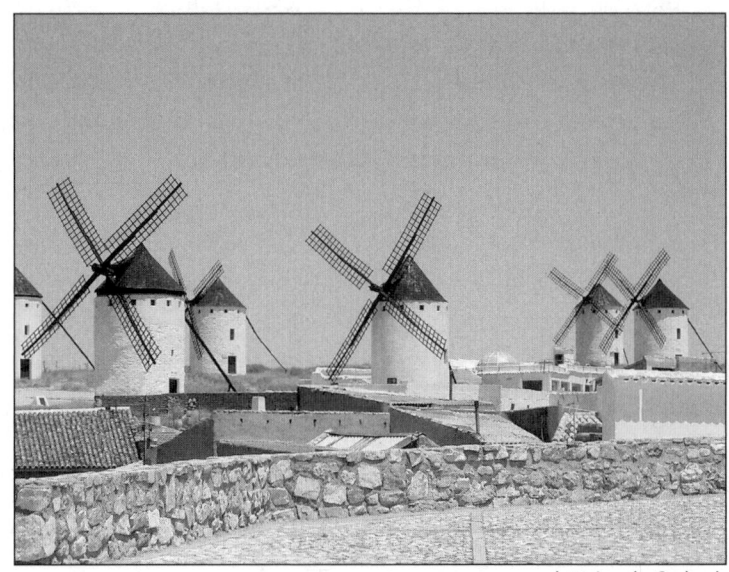

photo: Lourdes Cardenal

Campo de Criptana Molinos de Viento (Spain)
Classic Spanish windmills

Appendix I.

Of the Good Fortune Which the Valiant Don Quixote had in the Terrible and Undreamt-Of Adventure of the Windmills...

At this point they came in sight of thirty forty windmills that there are on plain, and as soon as Don Quixote saw them he said to his squire, "Fortune is arranging matters for us better than we could have shaped our desires ourselves, for look there, friend Sancho Panza, where thirty or more monstrous giants present themselves, all of whom I mean to engage in battle and slay, and with whose spoils we shall begin to make our fortunes; for this is righteous warfare, and it is God's good service to sweep so evil a breed from off the face of the earth."

"What giants?" said Sancho Panza.

"Those thou seest there," answered his master, "with the long arms, and some have them nearly two leagues long."

"Look, your worship," said Sancho; "what we see there are not giants but windmills, and what seem to be their arms are the sails that turned by the wind make the millstone go."

"It is easy to see," replied Don Quixote, "that thou art not used to this business of adventures; those are giants; and if thou art afraid, away with thee out of this and betake thyself to prayer while I engage them in fierce and unequal combat."

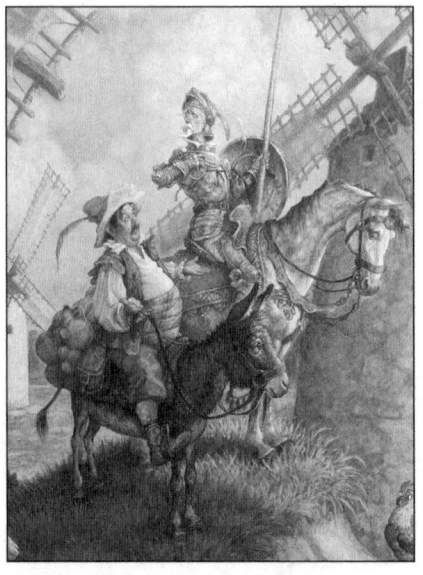

So saying, he gave the spur to his steed Rocinante, heedless of the cries his squire Sancho sent after him, warning him that most certainly they were windmills and not giants he was going to attack. He, however, was so positive they were giants that he neither heard the cries of Sancho, nor perceived, near as he was, what they were, but made at them shouting, "Fly not, cowards and vile beings, for a single knight attacks you."

A slight breeze at this moment sprang up, and the great sails began to move, seeing which Don Quixote exclaimed, "Though ye flourish more arms than the giant Briareus, ye have to reckon with me." So saying, and commending himself with all his heart to his lady Dulcinea, imploring her to support him in such a peril, with lance in rest and covered by his buckler, he charged at Rocinante's fullest gallop and fell upon the first mill that stood in front of him; but as he drove his lance-point into the sail the wind whirled it round with such force that it shivered the lance to pieces, sweeping with it horse and rider, who went rolling over on the plain, in a sorry condition.

Sancho hastened to his assistance as fast as his ass could go, and when he came up found him unable to move, with such a shock had Rocinante fallen with him. "God bless me!" said Sancho, "did I not tell your worship to mind what you were about, for they were only windmills? And no one could have made any mistake about it but one who had something of the same kind in his head."

"Hush, friend Sancho," replied Don Quixote, "the fortunes of war more than any other are liable to frequent fluctuations...

From *Don Quixote*, by Miguel de Cervantes. (Translated by John Ormsby. *www.manybooks.net*) p. 58

Letter to the President of the United States from Dr. Warren Levin

President Barack H. Obama
The White House
Washington, D.C.

April 20, 2009

Mr. President:

As a Fellow of the American Academy of Environmental Medicine, I was overjoyed by your campaign promises for a change in the USA's environmental stance. I am even more delighted by the actual changes already underway. Please, Stay the Course. What gives me the temerity to address a letter to the President is my standing in the community of Complementary Alternative Medicine [CAM]. I opened the first Holistic Health Center in NYC in 1974, and successfully fought against the suppression of my specialty by the NY State Office of Professional Misconduct. During that 14 year battle, I had great support from Berkley Bedell, Orin Hatch, Dan Burton and others on the Hill. I am on a first-name basis with most of the experts at your recent hearings on CAM, and I recently accepted the position of Chairman of Biomedical Education for a newly formed Northern Virginia chapter of the National Autism Association, a 501C-3 Foundation.

I am writing today because, in my fiftieth year of practice, I find myself at the center of three major "Controversies" in American Medicine. The federal government is right there with me, and it seems that neither of us has been able to effect the changes necessary. Although my desire and intent are strong, I certainly don't have the power, while the government appears to lack the cohesiveness between different offices needed to exert their combined influence on these areas of controversy:

1. Mercury and Fluorides in Dentistry
2. The alarming rise in Autism
3. Endemic Lyme disease.

These are entwined with one another, causally and therapeutically, and more importantly, **they suffer from the same underlying obstruction to change in their respective paradigms for diagnosis and treatment.** That blockage is the true subject of my letter. Truly, all progress in medical paradigms stems from Heresy, from holding opinions which are at variance with accepted beliefs!

Like it or not, we are today a litigious society, and the threat of lawsuits against the standard-bearers of the *status quo* makes it almost impossible to expect a change to take place voluntarily. For example:

1. The FDA has ignored rulings from the courts and instructions from the legislatures, with regard to publishing the scientific *proof* of the toxicity of mercury and fluoride. If they were to appropriately protect the public and announce the elimination of both of these substances from dental offices and public water supplies, the legal eagles

who specialize in *post facto* actions would have a field day, because **the science is compelling, it has been known for a long time, and the effects are actionable.**

2. The *status quo* in autism holds that this problem is incurable, and can only be dealt with by "rehabilitating" the various external expressions of the problem: speech, hearing, vision and musculoskeletal issues. What is totally ignored is the biochemistry of the brain, which must be diagnosed and individually addressed before full rehab can be accomplished. I am enclosing two DVD's showing recoveries based on such an approach, yet the centers for Pediatric Neurology have continued to ignore them for over a decade. Parents of these kids have spent a fortune trying to create a home environment to help them cope with their limitations, **whereas proper treatment allows the vast majority of them to rejoin the world.** If the major pediatric associations would change their opinions and accept the effective biochemical treatment of autism, many will attempt to exact retribution from the Authorities, because the science is compelling, it has been known for a long time, and the effects are actionable.

3. With regard to Lyme disease, the Infectious Disease Society of America, creators of the "official" Guidelines to Diagnosis and Treatment of Lyme Disease, as posted on the website, *www.guidelines.gov,* have recently been sued by the Attorney General of the State of Connecticut for conflict of interest in the creation of that document. The panel has been disbanded, a new panel appointed, and hearings are underway. The new panelists have been sworn to freedom from conflict of interest and to the obligation to scientifically review all evidence that has

heretofore been arbitrarily rejected. All of this is under the watchful eye of a Professor of Medical Ethics. Nevertheless, a serious question remains as to whether the new panel's guidelines will leave the previous panel at risk for retaliation, because *the science is compelling, it has been known for a long time, and the effects are actionable.* In the meantime, as examples of the impact of the errors on quality of life, I have had two cases of ALS and one of MS, all of whom tested positive for Lyme by special testing, and all of whom made good to spectacular progress while on IV antibiotics. All of them were denied continuation of therapy by their insurance companies, because they "did not fit the guidelines," and all of them regressed when treatment was discontinued.

The common denominator that impedes the progress of science in our society is the certainty that lawsuits will follow any meaningful change in medical practice that does not represent a new technology, but merely a change in opinion.

I believe that the Federal Government should pass a broad amnesty bill, covering practitioners from lawsuits over changes in guidelines for diagnosis and treatment. Freed from that onerous burden, new committees will be free to create, and re-create, guidelines that can more truly represent current "Evidence-Based Medicine."

Sincerely,

Warren M. Levin, MD, FAAFP [ret] FAAEM, FACN

Appendix III.

Can Our Children Handle This???
48 Doses of 14 Vaccines
Before Age 6[178]

Birth	2 Months	4 Months	6 Months	7 Months
Hepatitis B	Diphtheria	Diphtheria	Diphtheria	Influenza
	Tetanus	Tetanus	Tetanus	
	Pertussis	Pertussis	Pertussis	
	Polio	Polio	Polio	
	HIB	HIB	PCV	
	PCV	PCV	Rotavirus	
	Rotavirus	Rotavirus	Hepatitis B	
	Hepatitis B		Influenza	

12-15 Mo.	18 Months	3 Years	4-6 Years
HIB	Diphtheria	Influenza	Diphtheria
PCV	Tetanus		Tetanus
Measles	Pertussis		Pertussis
Mumps	Hepatitis A		Polio
Rubella	Influenza		Measles
Varicella			Mumps
Hepatitis A			Rubella
			Varicella
			Hepatitis (2)

---

178   From the National Vaccine Information Center, NVIC

Vaccine Reactions: Mothers' Descriptions

High Fever (over 103° F) "His temperature was 105 degrees. I had to put cool towels on him to bring the fever down."

Skin (hives, rashes, swelling) "There was a big, hot swollen lump at the site of the shot that stayed for weeks."

High Pitched Screaming "It was a pain cry, a shrill scream and lasted for hours and nothing would help."

Collapse/Shock "She turned white with a blue tinge around her mouth and went completely limp."

Excessive Sleepiness "He passed out and we couldn't wake him to feed or do anything for over 12 hours."

Convulsion "Her eyes twitched, her chin trembled, her body went rigid and then would shake."

Brain Inflammation "He just laid in his crib with his eyes wide open then would arch his back and scream and go unconscious. Now he has seizures."

Behavior Changes "She won't sleep or eat. She throws herself down and screams for no reason. She was sweet and happy and is now out of control. She changed into a totally different child."

Mental/Physical Regression "My 18 month old son stopped talking and walking after those shots. He developed severe allergies, constant diarrhea, ear infections and was sick all the time."

Other reported vaccine reactions include loss of muscle control, paralysis, regressive autism, asthma, arthritis, blood disorders, diabetes, Guillain Barre Syndrome.

If your child's health deteriorates after vaccination, your child may be eligible for federal compensation. Vaccine reactions should be reported to the federal Vaccine Adverse Event Reporting System (VAERS) by calling 1-800-822-7967 and to NVIC's Vaccine Reaction Registry at *www.NVIC.org.*

Appendix IV.

Recommended Books and Websites

If I tried to list all the writers who infused their knowledge into the heart of this humble student of Don Quixote, I would never finish, and you wouldn't know where to start. Here are a few of my favorite works most specific to this book, plus a few must-read orthomolecular classics. They are in no order, except for how they sit on my shelves, from left to right. Maybe it would have been enough to show you a photograph.

Books

- Price, Weston, D.D.S. *Nutrition and Physical Degeneration.* Price-Pottenger Nutrition Foundation, 2008 (newest edition). (If you only read one nutrition book, this may be the best choice.)
- Williams, Roger J., Ph.D. *Biochemical Individuality: The Basis for the Genetotrophic Concept.* Connecticut: Keats Publishing, 1998. (A true classic, a necessity for understanding the paradigms of nutritional healing.)
- Hoffer, Abram, M.D., Ph.D., *Healing Children's Attention & Behavior Disorders.* Toronto: CCNM Press, 2005. (Dr. Hoffer writes in his Foreword: "If the program described here is followed by physicians and by patients and their families, there is no doubt that the vast majority of the children so treated will recover, and without the need for medication.")

- Hoffer, Abram, M.D., Ph.D. *Orthomolecular Treatment of Schizophrenia*. Los Angeles: Keats Publishing, 1999.
- Hoffer, Abram, M.D., Ph.D. and Walker, Morton, D.P.M. *Putting It All Together: The New Orthomolecular Nutrition*. Connecticut: Keats Publishing, 1996.
- Levy, Thomas, M.D. J.D. *Vitamin C, Infectious Diseases & Toxins: Curing the Incurable*. Xlibris, 2002.
- Emoto, Masaru. The Secret of Water For the Children of the World. Oregon: Atria Books, 2006. (All of Emoto's other books are recommended. I chose this one because it's written for children.)
- Pauling, Linus. *How to Live Longer and Feel Better*. Oregon State University Press, 2006. (This is the most recent edition of this classic book, by one of the most influential scientists of all time, the man who coined the word "orthomolecular.")
- Stone, Irwin. *The Healing Factor: Vitamin C Against Disease*. Grosset and Dunlap, 1972. (One of the classic books about vitamin C. It is now available for free downloading at *http://www.vitamincfoundation.org/stone.*)
- Holford, Patrick and Colson, Deborah. *Optimum Nutrition for Your Child's Mind: Maximize Your Child's Potential*. Celestial Arts, 2008. (An excellent companion book for the book now in your hands.)
- Pitchford, Paul. *Healing With Whole Foods: Asian Traditions and Modern Nutrition* — 3rd edition. North Atlantic Books, 2002.
- Brownstein, Dr. David. *Iodine: Why You Need It, Why You Can't Live Without It*. Medical Alternatives Press, 2008.
- Haas, Elson, M.D. *Staying Healthy with Nutrition: The Complete Guide to Nutritional Medicine*. Celestial Arts, 2006. (This book is written in the most readable style I've ever seen in a college textbook. Highly recommended for a layman wishing to learn about general nutrition.)
- Bergner, Paul. *The Healing Power of Minerals*. Prima Publishing, 1997.

- Erasmus, Udo. *Fats that Heal, Fats that Kill.* Alive Books, 1995.
- Edelman, Eva. *Natural Healing for Schizophrenia and Other Common Mental Disorders.* 3rd Edition. Borage Books, Oregon, 2001.
- Angell, Dr. Marcia. The Truth About the Drug Companies: How They Deceive Us and What To Do About It. Random House, 2004. Dr. Angell was editor in chief of the prestigious New England Journal of Medicine.

Websites

- *www.doctoryourself.com.* In my opinion, probably the best health site on the Web.
- *www.vitamincfoundation.org.* Starting with this site, you can spend a long time learning about the most important medicine in the world, vitamin C. Actually, I shouldn't call it a medicine, because then it could only be bought with a doctor's prescription. Site owner, Owen Fonorow, manages an excellent forum on the site.
- *www.imva.info.* The website of Mark Sircus, a leading, outspoken critic of the modern "health" system (Mark will be proud of me, when he sees that I wrote "health" with quotation marks. He's far more radical than I). Sircus teaches us about powerful, non-toxic treatments of disease.
- *www.pubmed.com.* The U.S. National Library of Medicine and Institutes of Health online library. References used in this book from this library contain a PMID number. Simply typing the number in the site's search column will get you to the study. It has always amazed me that I could sit in my little town and enter this immense library. What a privilege, and what a giant step for mankind!
- *www.autism.com.* The Autism Research Institute
- *www.ppnf.org.* Website of The Price-Pottenger Nutrition Foundation®. ("The goal of the Price-Pottenger Nutrition Foundation is

to advance and promote the principles of Dr. Price, Dr. Pottenger and like-minded researchers to uplift the human race to a higher physical, mental and spiritual consciousness. Among these principles is the conviction that the quality of the soil and the plant and animal kingdoms determine the physical foundation of mankind which in turn promotes and balances mental and spiritual growth.")

- *www.fluoridealert.org.* "Broadening public awareness about fluoride."

- *www.nvic.org* National Vaccine Information Center, "America's Vaccine Safety Watchdog." There are many radical anti-vaccine activists' sites on the Web, but this isn't one of them: "This website was created to provide you with the information you need to make an informed vaccination decision."

Note about photos: Images on pages 64, 93, and 276 are licensed under the terms of the Creative Commons, share and share alike with attribution license. See Wikipedia.org for details.

About the Author

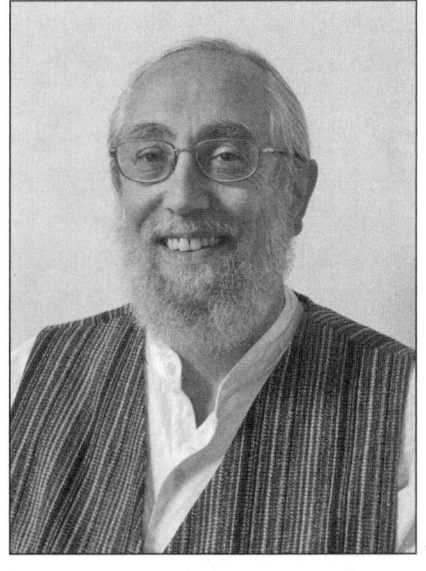

Dolev Reuven Gilmore, born in 1951, is the father of six children and grandfather of ~~10~~ ~~11~~ 12 (at printing time; more secrets may be revealed). That's a lot of qualification right there. He is also a born writer and speaker, passionate in expressing the ideas spawned by his deep thinking and caring spirit.

Having spent much of his life in field and forest, Gilmore, who grew up in Ohio, now lives in Israel. He farmed organically for a couple of decades, before a career change brought him to alternative medicine. For the past twelve years, Gilmore has immersed himself in studying and practicing nutrition, shiatsu and guided imagery, consulting, writing and teaching. In his words, "Studying the biochemical pathways of the human body and meeting people soul-to-soul in my clinic reveal the glory of God's creation to me, just like standing on a mountain and inhaling the beauty — something I've also done a lot of."

Gilmore lectures extensively, appearing before audiences ranging from sixth grade students to the elderly, from the general public to college students and health professionals. He visits the United States often, and is available for book promotion activities, interviews, lectures and consultations. The wonders of modern communications make radio interviews and phone consultations possible at any time, from anywhere in the world.

SPREAD THE WORD!

I hope that reading this book has been an enjoyable, eye-opening and mind-opening experience. I hope that you've begun to apply the information you've learned, and that you see your child blossoming. You will find, however, that your child's beyond-the-home environment is just the way it was last week. Birthday parties with sugar on top, candied friendships and sweet-toothed school lunches. Pediatricians peddling their traditional wares and shiny doctor-office pamphlets with no pictures of budding Don Quixotes on the covers. Media full of windmill chaff.

What to do? SPREAD THE WORD! Buy a bunch of copies of *Nutrition and Your Child's Soul* for your child's teachers and doctors, for your family and friends. Call us at 1-8777-CHILDREN (1-877-724-4537) for a discount rate. Or e-mail us at *info@ MindOppeningPublications.com* and tell us how many post cards with the cover image and ordering info you want to hand out. Show the book to your local health-food store owner, who will want to improve whole food and supplement sales by offering copies to their customers. When you're in the local library or bookstore, ask for the book, and they'll order it for their visitors. Bring the book to the attention of your local parent organizations, your book club and anyone you know who deals with children. If your child has special needs, you certainly know parents and caregivers in similar situations.

Keep in touch! Join the subscribers list at *www.dolevgilmore.com,* and we'll send you vital information about the latest research and clinical findings, as well as answers to subscribers' questions. (We won't bombard you with stuff – just a monthly or bimonthly update). Buy carefully chosen products on the website. We'll try to offer the best prices anywhere.

Ask health questions! You may want an opinion about the drug your doctor is prescribing, about the supplement schedule you're on, or other personal health issues. I'll be happy to respond quickly, if I can pull the answer out of my hat. If a question is more complicated, requiring information gathering, research, an involved written answer or a phone discussion, I'll suggest a fair payment for my time and expertise. E-mail me at dolev@dolevgilmore.com.

When you purchase *Nutrition and Your Child's Soul* directly from my website, you'll receive a choice of bonus offers, which will change from time to time: free shipping, a deep discount on a product, an e-book, etc.

Finally, everyone involved in Mind-Opening Publications and I wish all the best blessings for you and your family!

Index